Code Blue

Richard E. McDermott, Ph.D.
Kevin D. Stocks, Ph.D., CPA

Third Edition

W9-BFR-788

Traemus Books

2481 West 1425 South
Syracuse, Utah 84075
Phone: (801) 525-9643
Fax: (801) 773-7669
Email: kevin_stocks@byu.edu
Web Page: http://www.Traemus-Books.com

Web page: http://www.traemus-books.com

ISBN 0-9675072-0-0

To order additional copies go to web page: http://www.traemus-books.com And select **Order Copy Now** from bottom of home page or email Kevin_Stocks@byu.edu

Students: To download student questions and PowerPoint slides, or to ask the author a question, go to http://www.traemus-books.com and select **Student Resources** at the bottom of the home page.

Professors: To download lecture outlines, course outline guidelines, student questions, and PowerPoint slides, or to ask the author a question, go to http://www.traemus-books.com and select **Instructor Resources** at the bottom of the home page. To order answers to student questions, email author at kevin_stocks@byu.edu.. Include name, title, institution, department, mailing address, email address, phone, and course for which materials will be used.

Acknowledgments

Special thanks to the following who reviewed the book and provided helpful input:

Lavina Fielding Anderson, Edit Inc
Tara White, Editorial Assistant, Traemus Books
Elizabeth Dundas, Administrative Assistant, Traemus Books
Candadai Seshachari, Ph.D. Chairman of the English Department, Weber State University
Rick Fullmer, Administrator, University of Utah Medical Center
Robert Parker, former administrator, Brigham City Hospital, President EPIC
Monte Swain, Ph.D. Associate Professor of Accountancy, Brigham Young University

Preface

What you are about to read represents a new way of teaching technical material. As the approach is unorthodox, an explanation is warranted. The format chosen is that of a textbook-novel. It tells the story of a CPA who accepts a consulting job for a community hospital, a job that involves him in romance, mystery, murder, intrigue, and . . . *managed care!*

My primary purpose in selecting this format is *learning in context.* Many learners complain that traditional education fails to prepare them for the real world. In this textbook-novel, I discuss not only how to find the right answers but also how to identify the right questions. My experience has been that the second issue is often far more important than the first.

In a similar vein, the book stresses the principle that how a manager does something is often as important as what he or she does. Some managers fail even though they do the right thing— because they do it in the wrong way. It is not enough to be sincere; one must be right. It is not enough to be right; one must be effective!

Creativity is another topic that can best be covered in the format of a textbook-novel. *How does one apply old principles to a new environment? What process does one follow in breaking a complex consulting project into manageable tasks?*

Code Blue was written for anyone impacted by the cost of healthcare or interested in one "solution" that has been offered—a set of principles known as *managed care.* This audience certainly includes physicians, nurses, healthcare administrators, accountants, personnel directors and other executives of businesses that pay that cost through health insurance premiums.

In a recent *Fortune Magazine* poll, nearly two out of three CEOs called skyrocketing medical costs one of the most important problems facing American corporations. One-third of those surveyed stated that healthcare costs are the single biggest problem they would face this decade. The United States currently spends more than $1 trillion for healthcare. Projections indicate this figure will double within the next decade.

Code Blue also contains technical material for the accounting student who is interested in learning more about service industry or healthcare cost accounting. It has been three decades since the number of service-industry jobs in the United States bypassed those in manufacturing. Still, accounting textbooks continue to emphasize traditional manufacturing cost accounting while neglecting or even ignoring the service industry.

Technical supplements, found in the appendix, illustrate the concepts taught, explain service industry cost accounting and contrast it with manufacturing accounting. This material is not essential to the story line and can be skipped by the more general reader. Questions for each chapter can be found on the author's web page: *http://www.traemus-books.com.*

As a boy, I lived on the shores of Lake Washington in the small community of Hunt's Point. Many homes have docks, and one of our neighbors bought an airplane boat—not a plane with floating pods, as one often sees in that part of the country, but a plane with a hull—like a boat!

The advantages of such a craft in the Pacific Northwest are not hard to imagine, but the vehicle had some drawbacks. Although it did things neither a boat nor airplane could do alone, it didn't always fly as well as a plane nor sail as well as a boat. This analogy has come to me as I've studied the art of fiction. I am a hospital administrator turned consultant as well as a professor of accounting and healthcare administration. In my formal training, I was taught expository writing. Fiction is obviously a different animal.

In a professional article, the author begins with an introductory statement: a thesis that is followed by an explanation and a summary. Organization is tight—redundancy is discouraged. In fiction, the author must have a story line that involves opposition. Characters must be interesting; and the plot must keep moving. Merging the objectives of these two writing styles is fun but challenging, especially when the purpose is to explain the technical principles of managed care, accounting, and finance.

A textbook-novel is not as easy to write as a textbook and may not be as action focused as a novel. On the other hand, a textbook-novel is more informative than many novels and is certainly more interesting—perhaps even more educational from the standpoint of context—than a textbook.

As the creator of Code Blue, my goal is to make learning easy by making it fun. It is up to you to determine how successful I was in achieving this objective.

Richard E. McDermott, Ph.D.
September 25, 2002

Table of Contents

Major Characters

Dr. Ashton Amos—President of the medical staff, board member, cardiac surgeon

Birdie Bankhead—Administrator's secretary

David Brannan—Chairman of the Board of Peter Brannan Community Hospital, son of James and Rachel Brannan, brother of Matt, English Professor

James Brannan—Wealthy hospital benefactor, son of Peter Brannan

Matt Brannan—Physician, son of James and Rachel Brannan, friend of Amy Castleton

Mike Brannan—First member of the Brannan clan to settle Park City, silver baron

Peter Brannan—Son of Mike Brannan and husband of Sara, hospital founder and benefactor

Rachel Brannan—Wife of James Brannan, mother of Matt and David Brannan

Sara Brannan—Wife of Peter Brannan, hospital founder

Amy Castleton—Daughter of Hap Castleton

Hap Castleton—Former administrator of Peter Brannan Community Hospital (PBCH)

Helen Castleton—Wife of Hap Castleton

Del Cluff—Budget Director

Irene Cowdrey—Professor of Human Resource Management, Weber State University

Tony Devecchi—Real estate developer and entrepreneur

Wes Douglas—Interim Administrator, Peter Brannan Community Hospital

Kayla Elmore—Accounts Receivable Clerk

Elizabeth Flannigan—Director of Nurses

Dr. Emil Flagg—Physician and board member

Thayne Ford—Newspaper Editor

June Hammer—Chief Dietitian

Logan Harker—Utah Healthcare Association director

Karisa Holyoak—Managing Partner, hospital CPA firm

David Hull—Administrator, Snowline Regional Medical Center

Helen Ingersol—Board Member

Dr. Herb Krimmel—Health Economist, University Hospital

Al Kuxhausen—FBI agent

Pete Lister—Director of Marketing, St. Matt's Hospital

Peter O'Malley—Sergeant, Park City Police Department

Martha Nelson—Paradigm Medical Systems accountant

Larry Ortega—Director of Reimbursement, University Hospital

Ryan Raymer—Chief Pharmacist

Susan Wycoff Raymer—Mother of Rob Raymer, sister of Edward Wycoff

Dr. Allison Richards—Medical Director, University Hospital

Parker Richards—New Assistant Administrator, Peter Brannan Community Hospital

Roger Selman—Hap Castleton's controller

Natalie Simpson—Acting Controller, Peter Brannan Community Hospital

Jerry Smith—FAA investigator

Charles Stoker—HMO Director, University Hospital

Hank Ulman—Self-appointed union steward

Sharon Ulman—Wife of Hank Ulman, daughter of Sharon Wycoff Raymer, half sister of Ryan Raymer

Jackson White—Architect

Hyrum Whittingham—President, Park City State Bank

Arnold Wilson—Vice President, Park City State Bank

Edward S. Wycoff—Chairman of the Finance Committee of Peter Brannan Community Hospital

Don Yanamura—Human Resources Director, Peter Brannan Community Hospital

Barry Zaugg—Underworld figure

All characters are fictional.

1

Trip to McCall

September 4, 1999—Salt Lake City International Airport

It was 7:30 a.m., and the shadows of the Wasatch Mountains blanketed runway three-four-left as a blue and white Cessna 340 pulled out of the hangar, rolled onto the taxiway, and stopped. The roar of the twin 335-horsepower engines severed the crisp morning air, resonating angrily off the metal buildings to the west. Inside the private aircraft, the pilot, Hap Castleton, pulled his flight plan from a dog-eared navigation book and studied it for the vectors that would take him to Twin Falls, Boise, and, finally, McCall, Idaho.

Hap had a broad, generous face, graying brown hair, and a large frame. Deep creases mapped a face that had weathered the storms of thirty years as administrator of a small hospital in Park City, Utah. Satisfied with the route, he gently nudged his traveling companion, Del Cluff, and then traced the route on the map with his index finger.

Cluff, a thin man with receding auburn hair, looked up from a journal on cost accounting. His rooster-like eyes pecked at the map momentarily. Nodding at Hap, he returned to his journal.

Hap had invited Cluff to discuss changes in the Finance Department. The board was pushing for a major hospital reorganization, and Finance was a good place to start. He folded the aviation map and placed it next to his seat. Picking up the mike, he contacted ground control.

"Salt Lake ground—Cessna two-six Charlie requests taxi to runway three-four-left."

"Cessna two-six Charlie—cleared to taxi."

Hap increased his throttle, turning the plane south on the taxiway that would lead him to the assigned runway. The morning air was cool and the takeoff would be smooth. He tuned the radio to 118.3—the Salt Lake tower.

"Cessna two-six-Charlie requests clearance for takeoff."

"Cessna two-six-Charlie cleared for takeoff. Fly heading 320, climb to 13,000 feet, contact departure on 124.3," was the tower's reply.

Hap felt the freedom surge deep within him as he released the brakes, pushed forward on the throttle, and began his takeoff roll. Flying and fishing were his favorite hobbies. Heavy responsibilities at Peter Brannan Community Hospital made it difficult to find time for either—but today, things would be different.

The plane accelerated. At 140 knots, he gently pulled back on the control yoke. With a soft thump, the wheels left the runway and the small plane lunged skyward. The plane climbed to 13,000 feet and turned onto its assigned vector of 320 degrees. Hap checked his airspeed, studied his altimeter and compass, and adjusted the trim. Satisfied the plane was on course, he turned his attention to his assistant controller.

Del Cluff had been with the hospital for nine months. A meticulous accountant, Del irritated Hap almost as much as he irritated hospital supervisors. It wasn't just the fact that he was a bean counter, although that didn't help. Why anyone would want to spend his day with his nose buried in a ledger puzzled Hap. It wasn't even the preference shown to Cluff by Edward Wycoff, chairman of the Finance Committee, although anyone who could get along with Wycoff was suspect in Hap's eyes. No— there was something more to it, something he couldn't quite put his finger on.

Grabbing a sack from under his seat, Hap nudged Del on the leg. "Something to eat?"

Cluff managed a nauseous smile. Pointing to his stomach, he shook his head— negative. Hap grabbed a sandwich and took a generous bite, wiping his fingers on his flight suit.

Nervous stomach? He takes life too seriously.

The smell of eggs and mayonnaise filled the cockpit. Chewing ferociously now, he tuned the Nav Com radio to the next VOR. The plane crossed the first radio beacon.

✻   ✻   ✻

From the right seat, Del Cluff watched the pilot adjust the radio and wondered why he had accepted the invitation to fly with Hap Castleton. *Hope this yo-yo knows more about flying than he does about hospital administration . . .* Palms sweating, Cluff tightened his seat belt.

Hap's management style was an increasing source of irritation. He created more problems than Cluff and a small flock of hospital accountants could fix. Although his larger-than-life personality made him a hero to many of his employees, he was no hero to Cluff.

The situation at the hospital was desperate. There were rumors the board was planning a major change instigated by Edward Wycoff, finance committee chairman. Wycoff had been snooping around the Finance Department, reviewing records and quietly interviewing select members of the staff.

The operation needed a good review, but Wycoff scared the wits out of most of the employees. Wycoff's efforts only made the situation worse. If the hospital were a patient, Cluff thought, it would be a Code Blue: a flat line—cardiac arrest victim.

Cluff folded his journal, sliding it under his seat, and retrieved the navigation map. He studied it, then squinted nervously at the inhospitable terrain below. To the north lay Mount Ben Lomond, capped with snow from a storm that had moved through the Rocky Mountains two days earlier.

To the east were the cliffs of the rugged Wasatch Range, thrust high by a catastrophic rending millennia ago. To the west, the waters of the Great Salt Lake reflected the purple mountains of Antelope Island. Cluff shivered involuntarily. Folding the map, he returned it to the pocket by Hap's seat.

"Heard the rumors about Selman?" Hap asked, the irritation in his voice sawing the cold morning air. "Board's pushing for a change—Wycoff plans on firing him

Monday." Hap worked his jaw—his habit when irritated. "As soon as Selman's gone, Wycoff wants to install you as controller."

Cluff's eyes, a good barometer to his emotions, jumped in surprise. Cluff would welcome Roger Selman's dismissal—the two had frequently been at loggerheads. He would even welcome the opportunity to run things his way, but he wasn't entirely sure the promotion would be up—*it might be out.* It had been clear to Del from day one that Selman's position was dangerously close to the edge. Del said nothing while Hap struggled with his anger.

"Accept the job and you'll get two new responsibilities." His words were short and clipped. "The first is budget director—Wycoff wants $3 million cut from the budget—I want you to oppose him."

Fat chance! Cluff thought. *Half of our vendors have us on a cash-only basis; we aren't even sure we can meet payroll.* This wasn't the first time Hap had locked horns with Wycoff—he had no ally in Del Cluff.

"The second . . .?" Cluff asked.

"Project coordinator for a new cost accounting system." The yoke of the small aircraft started to pull. Hap adjusted the trim.

"Six months ago I asked the auditors to take a look at the operation, see if they could propose something. Insurance companies are killing us. The board isn't going to allow me to bid on another HMO[1] contract until we have a handle on the cost of our services."

Cluff's eyes narrowed with approval. He smiled. "Our auditors have been after Selman for a year to get a system up and running. They think this should be our number one priority."

Hap nodded decisively. "It's now *your* number one priority. Wycoff's hired a CPA, a fellow by the name of Wes Douglas, to serve as a consultant on the project. Wycoff wrote a memo to him—read it."

Cluff smirked sarcastically. He'd seen the memo. Wes was an eastern accountant and knew nothing about rural hospitals. He'd be more trouble than he was worth.

Earlier that morning, Hap received a briefing at the weather desk. An unstable air mass with high moisture content from Canada was moving into the state and was being lifted high by the steep terrain of the Rocky Mountains. Severe thunderstorms were probable.

Hap studied a dark bank of cumulus clouds at twelve o'clock. On his present vector he'd hit the storm head-on. He fished in his shirt pocket for a note card, then pointed to a dusty manual on the floor.

"I need a radio frequency—Twin Falls localizer. Think the frequency is 122.4 but I'm not . . ."

Hap aborted the sentence. Mouth wide open, he glanced at his instrument panel, then gaped out the window. His expression changed from disbelief to terror.

A cold wave of anxiety engulfed Cluff. "What's wrong?"

As Hap replied the color drained from his face. "The right engine—"

---

[1] Medical and accounting terms used in this story are defined in Appendix Two, *Medical, Economic, and Accounting Terms*

A thin ribbon of blue smoke was trailing from the engine. Hap reached for the throttle. Before he could reduce power, however, a violent explosion rocked the plane, whipping Cluff's head so violently he could taste the pain.

Hap grabbed the yoke in an attempt to regain control of the aircraft.

"Fire!" Cluff screamed.

The plane banked dangerously while Hap reached for the radio.

"Mayday, Mayday, Mayday," he shouted "Cessna two-six Charlie. Lost an engine . . . on-board fire." He glanced at the altimeter "Descending out of one-two-niner. Request immediate vector—emergency landing!"

One engine dead, the Cessna pulled right, the centrifugal force created by the right engine threatening to pull the plane into a flat spin. A spin would give the aircraft the flight characteristics of a pitching anvil—no lift; just spin, speed, and mass. "Can't hold it!" He shouted, jamming his foot into the left rudder.

"Throttle back . . . cut the left engine!" Hap said to himself.

He lunged for the throttles, inadvertently cutting power to both engines. The plane shuddered—then dropped like a roller coaster. Unable to pull it out, Hap wrapped both arms around the control yoke. The veins in his neck protruded like steel cables as he pulled with all the strength of his 250-pound frame.

At 280 knots, the burning engine disintegrated, its broken cowling ripping the horizontal stabilizer from the tail as it cleared the aircraft. A side window blew out.

Cluff grabbed for something to hold on to—the ride down got rougher still.

Still struggling with the yoke, Hap turned the plane north in the direction of Highway 82. It was apparent from the glide slope they wouldn't make it. An alarm sounded—red and amber lights exploded on the instrument panel.

Heart pounding like a sledgehammer, Cluff gaped at the rapidly approaching terrain below. To the west were homes and apartment complexes. To the east nothing but the foothills of the jagged Wasatch Mountains. Directly in front of the plane lay a freshly harvested hay field.

A farmer observing the plummeting aircraft jumped from his tractor and ran for cover. Cluff's eyes desperately drank every detail of the approaching terrain as he searched for a way out.

The hayfield was flat—but too short for a landing. At the far end was an elementary school. Children were already playing in the yard, waiting for the morning bell to ring. Cluff pointed. "Try for the field!"

"We'll hit the kids."

"They'll scatter."

"Can't chance it . . ."

This idiot's gonna kill us!

Hap banked the plane east toward the foothills. Completing the turn, he dropped his flaps. An alarm sounded—the landing gear wasn't down!

Rough terrain—bring her in on her belly. Hap turned off the electrical system. The blue and white Cessna, both engines silent, skimmed a row of cottonwood trees. The yoke was heavy and unresponsive. As Cluff screamed in terror, Hap Castleton tightened his harness and braced himself for the crash.

2

The Board

Edward Wycoff arrived at the hospital at 6:30 on Monday morning—a half hour before an emergency meeting of the board of trustees. Exploding down the hallway, he ignored the greetings of the housekeepers. Without breaking stride, he threw open the large walnut doors of the boardroom and switched on the lights.

Throwing his briefcase on a small telephone desk, he inspected the room. A retired officer in the Army Reserves, he knew how to conduct an inspection. Pity the employee who failed to meet his expectations.

Consistent with his instructions, the housekeeper had vacuumed the carpets and polished the conference room table until it shone like the brass on his colonel's uniform. He picked up the phone and punched in the extension of the Dietary Department. The Dietary Director answered.

"Wycoff here!" His commanding tone never failed to catch an employee's attention. "I ordered breakfast for the board!"

Telephone in one hand, the chief dietitian motioned frantically at a transportation aide. The aide clumsily shoved the heavy cart toward a service elevator. "Cart's on the way, Mr. Wycoff. Would've been there earlier but—"

Wycoff hung up, unwilling to grant her the satisfaction of an explanation. For a moment, the room was silent as he admired his reflection on the marble surface of the boardroom table. His most distinguishing features were his eyes—small and deliberate, the color of chipped ice. As always, he was unstirred by currents of self-doubt. *Hesitate—even for a moment—and you'll lose. Compassion now would only dull the victory . . .*

✳ ✳ ✳

Dr. Ashton Amos stuck his head through the door. At six-foot-one, he looked more like a basketball player than the newly elected president of the medical staff. His boyish mannerisms—coordinated awkwardness and a grin—made him popular with employees and physicians alike—a characteristic Wycoff could capitalize on.

Weariness from a twenty-eight-hour shift in the Coronary Care Unit lined Dr. Amos' voice. "Got your message," he said. "Just finished rounds . . . can talk now if you'd like."

Wycoff nodded. "Come in," he said evenly.

Dr. Amos crossed the room, seating himself in a large leather chair across from Wycoff. Retrieving a clean handkerchief from his pocket, he wiped his face and then blew his nose.

"Spent the night at the hospital?" Wycoff asked.

The doctor's mouth drew into a grim line. He nodded. "Fifty-one-year-old patient." Removing his glasses, he slowly massaged his eyes. "Double bypass—complications." Wycoff was unmoved; he'd give no sympathy.

"Any word on Hap's accident?" Amos asked, changing the subject.

Wycoff shook his head. "The plane hit fifty feet below the foothill summit. Sheriff thinks they were trying to reach Mountain Road. An FAA team arrived Saturday—I don't think they know anything yet. Have you heard anything about Hap's funeral?"

"It's scheduled for next Monday—noon. I've canceled surgery."

Wycoff nodded. "What about Cluff? What's the report?" Dr. Amos had emergency call the night Cluff had been brought in.

"Life-flighted to University Hospital. Called his attending physician this morning. Listed as critical—they think he'll make it." The room was silent as Wycoff digested the information. The young doctor knew that he hadn't been summoned to report on Cluff. Unless Cluff's services were needed again—a dubious probability considering the massive injuries he sustained from the crash—Wycoff would give no further thought to Cluff's welfare.

"What's the board going to do about a new administrator?"

Wycoff pursed his lips as though it was the first time he'd considered the question. "It's been a difficult weekend for me," he began, mouthing the words he had carefully rehearsed earlier. "Hap and I disagreed—disagreed often," he said, nodding in agreement with himself. "Still, I had a great deal of respect for the man."

Wycoff was lying, of course. He didn't think Amos would know the difference. He was wrong.

Wycoff steepled his fingers, a gesture of authority he'd used with good effect on Wall Street. "I've spent the past two days agonizing over the best course of action for the hospital." He hesitated. "I have a proposal, but I'm not sure if the board will buy it."

An ingratiating smile played on his lips as he leaned forward. He pointed an arthritic finger at Amos. "I need someone with your prestige to explain it to them," Wycoff continued. "Someone they respect, someone they'll listen to!"

Everyone knew how patronizing Wycoff could be when he wanted something. Dr. Amos felt vaguely nauseous.

"It's been my experience that the board rarely turns down one of your recommendations," Dr. Amos replied, his face masked and expressionless.

"It's essential the board pick the right man to replace Hap," Wycoff continued. "That won't happen overnight. While we're interviewing candidates, we need an interim administrator."

Amos nodded, his face softening with relief. There were rumors Wycoff had planned to bring one of his hired guns in from New York to operate the hospital.

"Someone strong enough," Wycoff continued, "to fully implement managed care at Peter Brannan Community Hospital."

A temporary appointment would be okay, thought Dr. Amos. *It would give the hospital an opportunity to recover from the death of Hap while providing the time to organize the medical staff, in the event Wycoff still plans a coup.*

"Any candidates?" Dr. Amos asked, interest written clearly on his face.

"None of our department heads are qualified. We need a *financial* person," Wycoff said with emphasis. Someone who can address the problems we're having with prospective payment systems!"

Ah! Prospective payment! thought Dr. Amos. *A term used often these days.* It referred to a practice insurance companies had adopted of negotiating fixed price contracts for healthcare in advance of treatment. The intent was to shift economic risk from the payer to the hospital. It was meeting its purpose. Since its adoption by Medicare and a host of insurance companies, life had grown increasingly difficult for physicians and administrators.

Someone would have to address the problem, but Amos himself was at a loss to identify a candidate. The physicians were too poorly organized, and the young MBAs didn't understand the uniqueness of healthcare.

"Suggestions?" he asked.

"There's a new CPA in the community—a fellow by the name of Wes Douglas. The hospital hired him a few weeks ago for a consulting project. He has no preconceived notions and isn't involved with hospital politics."

Interim appointment . . . he might be okay, Amos thought. "Does he have the time?" he asked.

Wycoff nodded. "I phoned him last night. He's still building his practice. He's not only got the time; he needs the money."

Amos smiled. Wycoff could always identify a person's Achilles heel—he obviously had found Wes's. Amos rose thoughtfully and walked to the French doors overlooking the west patio. It was 7:00 a.m. and the morning shift was arriving. Mary Hammond was parking her car. A widow with six children, she worked as a clerk in the operating room. Retrieving her lunch from the front seat of a battered 1972 Honda, she hurried to the employees' entrance.

As Dr. Amos watched her, he reflected on the hospital's financial problems and the effect closure would have on the employees who depended on it for their livelihood. He turned to Wycoff. "I don't have any better ideas," he said with a shrug. "I'll support the recommendation. Of course, I can't speak for the other members of the board."

3

A Change of Seasons

Thirty-one-year-old Wes Douglas stepped from his car to the sidewalk. He stretched the knots out of his back as he surveyed the wooded grounds of Peter Brannan Community Hospital. The change of seasons had come suddenly this year. Colorful leaves blanketed the lawn like the patchwork quilts sold in the gift shop. Wes enjoyed all the seasons, but fall—the season of change—was his favorite. Watching a gust of wind stir the leaves, he pondered the impending changes that awaited his career as he prepared for his interview.

Hap Castleton had stood with him here, on a hot day in mid-September, and explained the crisis that motivated the hospital to hire Wes as a consultant. The board of trustees was concerned about the hospital's lack of financial controls under the new prospective payment systems adopted by many insurance programs, including Medicare and Medicaid. Hap asked Wes to design a cost accounting system to provide the data necessary to bid and manage prospective payment system contracts. For the consulting engagement, Wes would receive $50,000.

Wes had spent less than a week working with Hap on the project but was impressed by his energy and enthusiasm. Hap was an extrovert. His expressive style won the approval of employees and medical staff. Hap understood people and was a master at hospital politics. He was weak, however, in operations—at least according to Edward Wycoff.

Wes, on the other hand, understood finance and operations. At Lytle, Moorehouse and Butler, his former CPA firm, he had consulted with a host of manufacturing firms and assisted in the design of financial control systems—systems designed to restore profitability in an increasingly competitive international manufacturing environment.

Wes had a mind for detail, and he was a workaholic. Long after the staff went home, Wes pored over production reports and product flow diagrams, identifying inefficiencies that slowed production and increased cost.

Wycoff had picked up on the difference between Wes and Hap during Wes's first interview. The two had finished dinner and retired to a richly paneled lounge on the second floor of the Yarrow Inn.

"I want to tell you a story," Wycoff said, lighting a cigar as he settled into a large wing back chair. "One of my neighbors in New York, a fellow by the name of Eric Rose, was vice president of General Electric. When he retired, he had thirty years with the company. Four of the company's officers retired at the same time—three vice presidents and a director. Thanks to General Electric's generous stock-option program, they retired wealthy, sure of their business ability.

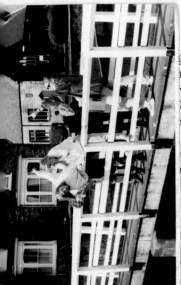

glasses, placing them on a table by his chair. "Wes, sixty-
[...]ing. After short vacations, Eric and the three other officers
[...]wn. They had a lot of confidence."

[...]or emphasis. "Within three years, each lost his investment!
[...]ed into personal bankruptcy. For a long time, I wondered
[...] billion-dollar corporation couldn't make a success of their
[...]d. "Want to guess why they failed?"

[...]erience in a new industry?"

[...] I think the main reason was that they no longer had the
[...]eam. At General Electric, the VP of research had the VP of
[...]at he had to develop products that would sell. The VP of
[...] of the VP of engineering to make sure he wouldn't pre-sell
[...]ilt."

[...]VP had the VP of finance looking over his shoulders,
[...]st so his products could be priced at a level the customer
[...]ance, of course, had the other three VPs to remind him that
without Marketing, Engineering, and Research, he wouldn't have a job!"

Wycoff smiled reproachfully. "My friends failed because they chose partners that
were just like them—not just in experience, but also in aptitude."

"You're saying they failed to select people who could compensate for their blind
spots," Wes affirmed.

Wycoff's eyes danced approvingly. "That's right. And that's why I'm interested
in your experience." Wycoff pressed his lips shut as he studied the young consultant.
"I think you could help us with more than the design of a new accounting system. I'd
like to see you serve as a permanent consultant to the board in financial and operational
controls."

Wycoff leaned forward as though he was going to share a secret. "I'll admit
Castleton is great with people," he whispered, "but he's poor with details, and he lacks
a *financial perspective*. He knows the politics of the hospital, but you understand
management and cost control. *Alone*, neither of you could run a business as complex as
Peter Brannan Community Hospital. As a *team*, however, I think you'd be
unbeatable!"

Standing now on the front lawn of Peter Brannan Community Hospital, two weeks
after that initial conversation, Wes realized that Wycoff's ideas were no longer valid.
Hap was gone, and without him there was no team. Without a team there would be no
consulting contract.

Losing the job would be a bitter experience. Wes totaled his outstanding financial
obligations—*$1,000 for office rent, $600 for part-time secretarial services, and a
payment of $1,000 or so on a $24,000 hospital bill*. The latter was his largest
obligation. The collections department at Community Hospital in Hartford was less
than sympathetic.

Nine months earlier he was involved in a serious automobile accident. His
insurance only paid a small portion of the hospital bill. He signed a note for the
balance. Since coming to Park City he had been unable to make regular payments, and
the hospital's business office manager was threatening to turn it over to an attorney.

Wes bent forward in an effort to relieve the throbbing pain in his back. Muscle spasms caused by stress, aggravated the problem—and today he was stressed! Gently stretching backwards now, he noted there was less numbness in his left leg than a month ago—a good sign. If only he could say the same thing for the numbness in his soul.

Flexing his knees so as not to bend or twist, Wes Douglas gently stooped to pick up his briefcase. Forcing a smile, he bravely crossed the lawn, entering through the large brass doors of the visitors' lobby.

* * *

A row of wooden chairs with straight, upright backs stood sentry at the entrance to the lobby, and the scent of ethyl alcohol and cresyl violet seeped into the hall from the small laboratory on the first floor. Wes's leather-soled shoes squeaked on the highly waxed linoleum floor as he crossed the lobby to the information desk. He spoke briefly with the receptionist, then went directly to Administration where Birdie Bankhead, secretary to the administrator, greeted him.

Birdie, a fifty-six-year-old divorcee with two grandchildren and a poodle, had worked at the hospital as long as Hap. With red eyes and splotched cheeks, she looked up from the newspaper. Hap Castleton's picture was on the front page.

"I'm Mr. Douglas," he said, "I'm here to meet with the board."

Birdie nodded in recognition. "They're running a few minutes late. Would you like some coffee or juice while you wait?"

"No, I'm fine."

Birdie wiped the corners of her eyes with a handkerchief. She opened her purse and retrieved a small makeup compact. "Sorry," she said as she excused herself. "It's been a difficult morning for all of us. I'll be gone for a few minutes. If you need anything, Mary Anne in the next office can help."

Wes nodded understandingly as Birdie left. Hands in his pockets, he scanned the room. The office was fourteen feet square and served as the reception area for the administrator's office and the boardroom. The door to the boardroom was slightly ajar, and from the conversation that drifted through the door, he could tell the meeting was winding down. A woman was speaking.

"I'm not sure there's anything we can do but what you suggest," she said. "While I don't like it, you've convinced me it's our best alternative."

"All in favor?" a male voice said. There was a volley of "I's."

"Those opposed?" There was one vigorous voice of dissent.

* * *

The door to the boardroom opened wide, and Dr. Ashton Amos emerged, extending his hand in greeting. Wes shook it as the doctor apologized for the delay. "Hope you haven't been here long," he said. Wes shook his head no and Amos gestured for him to enter the boardroom. Inside, four members huddled in quiet conversation around a large conference table. Octagon in shape, it was cut from a one-inch slab of white Tennessee marble and rested solidly on a square platform of highly polished walnut. In the center stood an architect's model of the new hospital Hap Castleton had hoped to build—a project canceled three days before his death.

"I don't think you've met the entire board," Amos said. This is David Brannan, chairman of the board." Dr. Amos pointed to a well-dressed man in his early thirties. "From his last name, you can tell his family has played an important role in the history of the hospital." Wes smiled in acknowledgment, while Brannan stood and shook his hand.

"Next to David is Dr. Emil Flagg, the Medical Staff's representative on the board." Dr. Flagg, a pathologist in his early sixties, had a dyspeptic smile and smelled vaguely of formaldehyde. Stretch wrinkles radiated from the single button of an enormous white lab coat that struggled to corral his rotund torso. Flagg glowered as he scrutinized Wes from head to toe, then nodded abruptly.

"Helen Ingersol, president of Ingersol Construction is next. This is Helen's first meeting with the committee." Helen Ingersol, a strong administrative type with short brown hair, and blue eyes that flashed intelligence, smiled acknowledgement.

"And last, but not least, is Ed Wycoff. You already know Mr. Wycoff." Wycoff motioned for Wes to take the chair next to him.

"The tragic events of the weekend have forced us to make some difficult decisions," Wycoff said, his lips compressing into a cold, thin line. "As these involve your consulting contract, we felt we should involve you in the discussion."

Wycoff paused. "Before addressing that issue, however, we have one other item of business. Dr. Amos, would you invite Roger Selman in?" As Amos left the room, Wycoff turned to Wes. "Roger is the hospital controller."

Wes had worked for his grandfather the summer before college, herding sheep in the mountains high above his Wyoming ranch. Sometimes dark thunderheads appeared on the horizon, churning their way toward the summer pasture. Even though the air was deathly still, uneasiness always proceeded the pyrotechnics soon to come. That same atmosphere filled the room as Amos returned with Selman. Both men took their seats—Brannan next to Wycoff and Selman at the end.

Except for the drumming of Wycoff's fingers on the cold marble table, the room was silent. Wycoff carefully studied the concerned face of each board member. Satisfied he had their attention, he removed the hospital's financial report from a manila folder and carefully placed it on the table. He gazed at it for a moment, withdrawing his hands for dramatic effect.

"Lady and gentlemen," he said, "Mr. Selman has provided us with an unusual document. In my twenty years as a financial analyst, I have never seen anything like it!" He paused for emphasis. "You are to be congratulated, Mr. Selman!"

Wycoff's sarcasm was not lost on Selman, who squirmed in his chair and smiled uncomfortably.

"Mr. Selman, when you joined the hospital five years ago, we had a successful business. No debts—a million dollars in the bank." Wycoff took a drink of ice water, then wiped his mouth with a handkerchief.

Beads of perspiration formed on Selman's forehead. With a beefy forefinger he tugged on his collar, loosening the knot of his necktie that seemed to tighten even as Wycoff spoke.

Wycoff's eyes narrowed. "The report given this morning shows a substantial reversal," he said glacially. Still staring at Selman, he methodically flipped—one by one—through the pages of the report.

"During the previous twelve months," he continued, "We generated a loss of $3 million. Monday morning, our borrowing reached *two million dollars,* taking us within one hundred thousand dollars of our credit limit. With less than one hundred fifty thousand dollars of cash in the bank, we are perilously close to not being able to make payroll. Why, Mr. Selman," he said with callous sarcasm, "you and your associates have taken us to the edge of bankruptcy!"

From the expression on their faces, it was apparent that the board was not comfortable with the acerbic approach Wycoff was taking. Still, no one spoke.

Roger Selman took a deep breath. "It's been a difficult year," he acknowledged nervously, "but I think the worst is behind us. Yes, we've had trouble with the accounting system, but we can fix it. That's why Wes Douglas is here, isn't it?"

Breaking the lock of Wycoff's gaze, Roger shot a plea for help to David Brannan who had always been more sympathetic than the rest. "Give me three or four months," he said, "and you'll see a dramatic reversal of our position."

Wycoff slammed the table. "We can't survive that long! For the past three years, we've seen a steady decline in financial strength. While we can't hold you solely responsible, your inability to provide cost information has significantly affected our ability to operate this facility."

Wycoff's voice lowered as he sighted in on Roger Selman for the final kill. "Mr. Selman," he said, "with the death of Hap Castleton, we have decided to reorganize the administrative council. As a part of the reorganization, we are asking for your resignation." Wycoff forced his lips into a glacial smile. "If you don't resign," he continued, "you will, of course, be terminated."

Selman gasped as if he had been hit in the abdomen. He scanned the faces of the board, searching for any indication of support—but none was offered. Denied a reprieve, he settled back in the large leather chair. In a minute or so, the tight lines around his mouth relaxed as fatigue replaced shock.

Roger Selman was sixty-two years old—and he was tired. He was tired of fighting Administration and the board. He was tired of operating a department with few resources, but most of all he was tired of the long hours it took to straighten out the problems created by well-meaning but inefficient Hap Castleton.

His emotions surprised him. He was no longer angry, he was relieved. *Without Wycoff, I might live another ten years. The money isn't that important. I can find another job; maybe I'll even start enjoying life again.*

Selman turned to Wycoff, who watched the transformation with quiet curiosity. Selman decided to give a speech he had rehearsed, but never before had courage to deliver.

"The world has changed, but the board is still living in the 1960s," he began. "Healthcare is no longer a charitable endeavor—it's a business. For five years I've told you we need a cost accounting system—something that will allow us to bid intelligently on prospective payment contracts.

"You've ignored me. At your direction, we've been bidding on fixed price contracts anyway—and we've bid wrong! Thanks to you, we don't even know where we're losing money.

Selman drew a bead on Wycoff. "It's the board's responsibility to provide direction and control. Mr. Wycoff, you have provided neither. You failed to act, and the hospital's reaped the consequences.

"The physicians complain about inefficiencies," Selman continued, turning to Flagg. "But most physicians haven't got a clue about what it takes to run a profitable hospital. The medical staff can't even agree on the most mundane matters.

"The hospital *is* in trouble," Selman continued. "But firing me isn't going to fix that. The operation needs to adapt, but I'm afraid that won't happen as long as you dinosaurs are in control." Wycoff sat up abruptly, insulted at Selman's description.

Roger Selman folded his papers and stuffed them into the large envelope he had carried into the meeting. He stood and shook his head in quiet disgust at Wycoff, then crossed the room. "Welcome to the twenty-first century," he said as he shut the massive walnut door behind him.

The room was silent as board members studied each other, uncertain how they felt about Wycoff's action—or Selman's response. Before they could react, Wycoff spoke.

"Mr. Douglas," he said, "the board has empowered me to offer you a contract to serve as interim administrator of Peter Brannan Community Hospital—just until we find a permanent replacement. We know you're not a hospital administrator, but you understand finance—which, for the moment, at least, is our most pressing need."

Wes looked up in surprise. *Interim administrator?* Unwilling to speak until he had thought the offer through, Wes studied the board members. In the two weeks Wes had worked with the hospital on the design of the new accounting system, he had lost much of his enthusiasm for Edward Wycoff. Working with him would be difficult.

On the other hand, Wes had consulted with small firms in trouble and had enjoyed the challenge. His practice was small, and he did have the time. If he did a good job, it might lead to future consulting jobs in the industry. Accepting the assignment would be a good way to become better known in the community.

Awkwardly, Wes cleared his throat. "If we can work out something financially, I think it might be an interesting project."

"We'll pay $5,000 a month for six months," Wycoff said.

Wes did the calculation in his head. "That's about $30 an hour. My consulting rate is four times that."

The lines deepened around Wycoff's mouth. He shook his head with firm determination. "The hospital's in financial difficulty, Wes. We can't afford that. Seven thousand a month is our best offer, guaranteed for six months if you do a good job—longer if it takes more time to get a permanent replacement."

Wes thought about his new accounting practice. He had only billed thirty hours last month. In a week or so he could finish up the current projects and sublet the office to save overhead. Once again, he turned the offer over in his mind. His eyes softened as he came to a decision. "I accept," he said.

Wycoff smiled smugly as he sank back into the large wingback chair. Expressions of the other board members ranged from happiness, to relief, to despair.

David Brannan broke the silence. "I don't mean to change the subject, Ed, but I have a meeting downtown in twenty minutes. Do we have enough cash to meet the payroll Friday?"

"Spoke with the business office last night." replied Wycoff. "They're expecting a $400,000 payment from Medicaid . . . should receive it by Wednesday. With that and the remaining line of credit, we should be able to squeak by."

"Any chance it won't be here in time?" Brannan queried.

"If it's not here by Wednesday, I'll drive to Salt Lake and walk the check through the Department of Social Services myself," Wycoff said. He had done this before.

"If payroll is covered, then I suggest we adjourn," said Brannan, smiling with relief. "Do I have a motion we adjourn?"

"I so move!" said Dr. Ashton Amos.

* * *

It was evening when Wes entered the administrator's office for the first time since assuming his interim post. He was surprised to see Hap's untouched books, journals, and memorabilia. He gazed at the personal items—family photos, a dusty rainbow trout, and a pair of running shoes—and remembered his last visit to the office. Hap's beaming personality had permeated the room like the rays of sun that had poured in through the French doors behind his desk.

The room was different today. The forest-green drapes were drawn, and except for the light from a small corner lamp, the office was dark and tomblike. Wes turned on the lights, opened the curtains, and settled into the large green armchair facing the desk.

The administrative wing was empty. He was grateful for the silence as he reflected on the events of the day. Had he participated in the discussions that led to the firing of Selman, Wes would have opposed it. Even if Selman was incompetent, he took knowledge that would have been helpful to a new administrator. After the meeting, Wycoff explained that the action was inevitable and that he had decided to spare Wes the task.

Although Wycoff's intent may have been good, it had clearly backfired. Selman was well liked; his dismissal, so soon after Hap's death, shocked and offended the employees. The hostility was more than evident at a meeting held later that morning when Wycoff introduced Wes as the interim administrator.

When Wycoff announced the termination of Selman, two female employees on the front row began crying, and a supervisor stormed from the meeting. Four department managers introduced themselves afterward in an attempt to be cordial, but it was apparent that most blamed Wes for the release of Selman. *If Wycoff had planned to set me up to fail, he couldn't have a done a better job*, Wes thought.

Wycoff was obviously not well tuned to the sensitivities of other people. The word on the street was that he was bright, but ruthless. Although this was a temporary position, Wes was beginning to realize the negative effect it might have on his fledgling CPA practice.

His thoughts were interrupted as Birdie Bankhead, the secretary to the administrator, entered the room. She carried a large yellow envelope. "I thought you'd left for the day," Wes said, looking up in surprise.

"I had, but our application for an accreditation visit has to be in Chicago by Friday."

Birdie's lips were drawn tight and Wes realized that she was struggling with some fairly strong emotions.

"If you'll sign the forms, I'll drop them by the post office tonight," she continued. She handed him the forms. He signed them and handed them back. Wes detected her animosity. *It wasn't there this morning before Roger Selman's dismissal.*

Birdie's eyes glistened as they caught the picture of Hap's family on the desk. "You'll want Hap's things out of his office. I'll remove them tomorrow," she said stiffly.

"There's no hurry," he said softly. "Let his family do it—at their convenience."

Birdie looked at him through the cobwebs of reddened eyes. She hadn't slept for two nights, or maybe she was still asleep; this past week had been a nightmare. From deep inside, a mournful sob shook her frame.

Wes stood up and took her hand. "Listen Birdie," he said. "I don't agree with everything that's gone on. This whole thing has been kind of precipitous. Let's not rush Hap's family. I can work around his things for a few days."

Observing his sensitivity, the lines around Birdie's eyes softened. *I wonder if he knows what he's got himself into?* Birdie didn't understand why the board hired someone with no experience to take the reigns from Hap. *Maybe he's been selected to take the fall—to deflect the blame from Wycoff and the board if the hospital folds.* Her sympathy increased as she contemplated the probable consequences for Mr. Wes Douglas, for the hospital, and for employees like herself.

She took a deep breath, releasing it slowly. "I'm sorry about the reception you received at the meeting," she said, beginning anew. "The employees are good people. They're still in shock over Hap's death, and now with the firing of Roger Selman—."

Wes nodded. "I understand," he said. "I'm not happy about the way things were handled today." He shrugged and smiled weakly. She smiled sadly in return.

"Is there anything I can do before leaving this evening?" she asked, pointing at the pile of mail and messages on his desk.

"I'm flying to Seattle to finish an assignment for a local firm," he said. "Watch over things while I'm gone."

"When will you be back?"

"I told the board I could start a week from Monday."

"There's a phone call from Wycoff that might change your plans." Birdie paused uncertainly, then crossed to his desk, where she tore a phone message from a notepad. "Wycoff called an hour ago," she said. "The bank has canceled the hospital's line of credit. He doesn't think the hospital can make payroll."

Wes was speechless. She continued.

"You should also look at this." She handed him the evening edition of the *Park City Sentinel.* The headline read:

Hospital Employees Threaten Walkout

Vote "no-confidence" on appointment of new administrator

Wes blinked, eyes wide with bafflement as he read the lead article. Removing his glasses, he rubbed his eyes, then stared out the French doors at the black storm clouds gathering to the east. Deep in thought, he waited more than a minute before breaking the silence.

"Cancel my flight," he said.

* * *

For a more detailed introduction to prospective payment systems and historical pricing issues, read Supplement One: Cost Accounting in Healthcare, which is found in Appendix One. This is recommended reading for medical and nursing students, as well as administrative and accounting students.

4

Resolve and Regret

Through an open window in his one room efficiency apartment, Wes listened to noises of the street below. A freight truck was backing into an alley, and someone was shouting instructions to the driver in Spanish. The freight dock for the hotel next door was directly beneath his window.

He rubbed his eyes and checked his alarm—5:00 a.m. The evening news had forecast stormy weather, and Wes smelled the rain before it hit the dusty asphalt below. A gusty wind snatched a newspaper high in the air above the alley. He heard distant thunder in the mountains.

Wes stumbled to his feet and shut the window. He returned to his bed. Sinking in the pillow, he took a deep breath, held it, and slowly released it. *If I could relax the muscles in my back, the pain might subside,* he thought. He eyed the medication on the nightstand, tempted for a moment to take another Percodan, then shook his head with firm resolve. *No more painkillers this morning. They'll cloud my mind. I need all the faculties I have to handle my second day.*

He gently straightened. It had been six months since his automobile accident, and this morning the pain in his lower back was as severe as the night he was pulled from the mangled wreckage of his automobile. He vaguely remembered being lowered onto an ambulance litter and then losing consciousness. A few minutes later, somewhere on the turnpike, he became aware of his surroundings. A paramedic was starting an IV, and someone was reading his vital signs over the radio to a nurse at the hospital.

"Kathryn? . . . Where is Kathryn?" he asked.

"It's going to be all right buddy," the paramedic answered.

The paramedic lied—nothing would ever be right again. Friends told him that time would soften the loss. Someday his life would make sense again—that had yet to happen. The only relief was the distraction of hard work—filling his time with so many activities he didn't have time to dwell on the past.

Even so, his mind burned with her memory. Rarely an hour passed he didn't think of Kathryn—her slender figure, twinkling green eyes—the impish look that played around her mouth just before he kissed her.

His friends were right, though. It was time to move on with his life, and this had been one of his motivations for leaving Maine. Often in the slumber of early morning, however, he returned to the evening of the accident. In that recurring nightmare he would feel the play of the steering wheel in his hands as his tires slipped on the wet pavement, the crushing impact of the crash; the blackness that blended the smells of burning rubber and gasoline with the pain; and the sound of the rain as it hit the oily asphalt below.

* * *

Wes's body was heavy with fatigue as he drove to work an hour later. To focus his thoughts, he reviewed the events of the previous day. At 1:00 p.m., after being introduced to the department heads, he met with Elizabeth Flannigan, the director of nursing.

Flannigan was a tough supervisor, especially where it came to issues of quality. She ran her department with a General Patton-like efficiency that won both affection and animosity from the medical staff. Sensing the concern of the board for the financial position of the hospital, Wes spent the first ten minutes quizzing her about her budgeting system, the procedures for staffing, and cost control. He asked if she had a contingency plan for staff reduction.

He shouldn't have done that—at least during their introductory meeting. The nursing staff was paranoid enough as it was. Alarmed, Elizabeth ran to Dr. Emil Flagg, who confronted Wes in his office, pouncing on him with the fury of a Rocky Mountain hailstorm.

"Hell-bound financiers like Wycoff are destroying healthcare!" Flagg shouted, his enormous fists smashing a stack of financial reports on Wes's desk. "Wycoff, that miserable miscreant, thinks he can run this place like a brokerage house. This isn't Wall Street, and our patients aren't stocks and bonds!"

The meeting lasted for an hour. Flagg was angry at managed care, insurance companies, paperwork, hospital administrators, and the other members of the board. Wes, in his eyes, was obviously one with Wycoff. Wes assured him that human factors would be considered in any reorganization. Flagg didn't believe it.

As his car pulled into the parking lot, Wes wondered if he had made a mistake accepting the position. He thought it over, then shook his head in dissent. *Negative thinking never solved anything. Besides, what are my alternatives? My practice hasn't exactly taken off—this town has too many public accountants. What else is there to do? I could crawl back to the managing partner at Lytle, Moorehouse, and Butler.* Wes chortled good-humoredly. He still remembered the shock on his arrogant supervisor's face the day he submitted his resignation. *"Well, I've nev-ah hea'd of such a thing,"* the smug New Englander had replied on hearing the news.

The decision's been made. Right or wrong, I'm in this up to my ears. The jobs of 200 employees depend on me. This place has been around for sixty-five years. It might fail eventually—but not during my watch!

* * *

"Good morning, Mr. Douglas!" A notably more chipper Birdie Bankhead looked up from her computer and smiled brightly. The puffiness was gone from her eyes, and her voice was as cheerful as the pink pantsuit she was wearing. Wes was grateful for the transformation.

He smiled and pointed good naturedly at his watch. "You're up early," he said.

"I had a ton of letters to finish before the phone starts ringing."

32

Birdie continued typing, then looked up with a start. "That reminds me," she said. "Hank Ulman, president of the Employees' Council, called me at home last night. He wants to meet with you—this morning, ten o'clock, downtown at the Pipe Fitters Union Hall. I wrote the address down." She reached for her purse. Retrieving a small notepad, she tore the message off and handed it to Wes. "Nine-twenty South Brannan Avenue," she said. "Small red building—second floor—just above the bakery."

His brows pulled into a scowl as he read the note. "Didn't know we had a union."

"Technically, we don't, although there's been talk of one since Wycoff threatened not to approve the salary budget. He wanted Hap to cut salaries across the board by 12 percent. The news leaked to the employees, and the television stations picked it up. It made quite a stir in the community. Guess it's surfacing again," she sniffed as she returned to her typing.

"Hank Ulman—" Wes said, thoughtfully turning the note over in his hand. "An employee of ours?"

Birdie nodded. "Works in the maintenance department. Moonlights part time as a mechanic for a flight service in Salt Lake City. He has the reputation as an iconoclast. Ran once for city council—American Socialist Party ticket. Got seven votes."

"Most of our employees ignored him. When Wycoff began involving himself in the operation of the hospital four or five months ago, however, Ulman got elected president of the Employee Council."

Quiet surprise registered in Wes's eyes. "What do you mean by—*Wycoff's involved in the operations of the hospital?*"

"He got the board to appoint him Director of the Budget," Birdie replied. "In theory, it's not a line position. Once he got control of the hospital's budget, however, even Hap had a hard time keeping him from directing the activities of our department heads. Hap planned on taking that function back. Before his death he got Wycoff to agree to transfer the title to Del Cluff."

Wes was silent as he reexamined the note. "Call Ulman," he said finally "and tell him there'll be no meeting, at least not at the Union Hall. Then arrange a session with our employees for 10:30. Ask scheduling to pull in all of our on-call nurses—I want as many of our full-time staff to attend as possible. I don't want the department heads there," Wes added, "just employees. I'll meet with the supervisors tomorrow."

Birdie wrote the instructions in her planner.

Energized by the completion of his first official act as administrator, Wes realized now that he was hungry. "Think I'll catch breakfast," he said brightly. "When I get back, let's meet to plan the rest of the day."

* * *

This was Wes's first visit to the cafeteria. An arrow pointed to the basement. Taking the marked exit, he plowed down the stairs, shaking hands with two physicians on the first landing. They requested a meeting with him at his earliest convenience. "Schedule it with Birdie," he replied cordially as he continued down the stairs.

Although the lobby was as cold and uninviting as a train station, he was pleasantly surprised to find the cafeteria warm and cheerful. Nothing fancy—if anything it was a little homespun—checkered red and white tablecloths and freshly painted yellow walls.

33

Canyon Elementary School had decorated the south wall with crayon drawings depicting brightly colored surgeons assisted by chalk-white nurses. The aroma of eggs, bacon, and coffee wafted from a spotless kitchen. A radio was playing country music, and the room hummed with the pleasant chatter of fifty or so employees and visitors.

Wes selected a tray and headed for the cafeteria line, confident few employees would recognize him as the new administrator. Thus far he had only been introduced to the supervisors. *A good chance for a little reconnaissance,* he thought, grabbing a packet of silverware.

Wes had a roommate in college, a law student, who told him once of a hospital malpractice suit his class had studied. The suit involved a physician who accidentally severed a carotid artery during surgery. For two days attorneys interviewed physicians and nursing personnel in detail. Frustrated at their inability to crack the case, they dispatched two law clerks to the hospital. Posing as visitors, the clerks spent three days in the cafeteria, drinking coffee and eavesdropping on the conversations of hospital employees. "When employees are together they like to talk," Wes's roommate had told him.

Within the security of the hospital's cafeteria they discussed the case, condemned the incompetence of the physician, and revealed ongoing complaints about his professionalism, and the failure of the medical staff and board to curtail his privileges.

Having learned far more from the prattle of the cafeteria than they would have gleaned in ten months of depositions, the attorneys quietly approached hospital administration with their newfound evidence. The hospital settled out of court for two million dollars.

Wes paid for breakfast and took a table near the center of the cafeteria, not far from a group of housekeepers who had seated themselves at a large round table. "Did ya hear they fired poor old Mister Selman?" a heavy woman in a blue housekeeping uniform said to her companions as she buttered a thick pancake. From a picture in the hospital newsletter, Wes recognized her as Betsy Flint, one of the hospital's longest-term employees.

"It was Wycoff that got him," replied a co-worker, a frail lady with a thin rooster nose. "Now Mr. Castleton's dead, Wycoff's going to have his evil way with the hospital," she prattled, pointing with her fork to a picture of the hospital on the wall.

"Doc Flagg said he's been pushing staffing cuts for three months now," Betsy said, her dark brown eyes turning bitter. "He'll have us all on unemployment if he gets his way," she replied, nodding ominously at the other employees at the table.

"He don't believe in unemployment insurance," another housekeeper said. "He'll have us on the street!"

"Hap would never have stood for that," Betsy said, her eyes widening with indignation. She took a hearty bite of her cheese omelet and then leaned forward conspiratorially. "Say, what's this new administrator like?"

"He's a real dandy," her companion replied, mirroring Betsy's facial expression. "Flagg says he's Wycoff's man—a guy from back east, a fancy finance fella. Doc says he doesn't know nothin' about hospitals."

A flash of alarm exploded across Betsy's portly face. "Good Jehosophat!" she said, rocking back in her cafeteria chair. Wes held his breath as the vintage chair—a survivor from the original hospital—groaned under her weight.

It held, but his eavesdropping was interrupted by the cafeteria intercom. Someone was paging the administrator on line four. Several employees scanned the cafeteria for a look at their new boss. Wes finished his breakfast while the interest died down. Then dropping his tray on a conveyor belt, he headed for a phone in the hall.

"Wes speaking," he said.

Birdie was on the other end, her voice registered concern. "I have Wycoff on the line. Told him you were unavailable. He insisted I track you down," she said.

Given what he'd learned about Wycoff's propensity to involve himself in operations, Wes had wondered how long it would take for him to call. He realized that if he were to be effective, he would have to impress Wycoff with one message: *The board establishes policy, raises capital, and hires and fires the CEO. Internal operations, however, are the sole responsibility of the hospital administrator.*

"Put Mr. Wycoff on," Wes said tersely.

The phone clicked. It was Wycoff.

"Wes, I saw the article in last night's paper. I'll be down in a few minutes to meet with the Employee Council. I've dealt with employee threats before—I'll nip this thing in the bud."

"Appreciate your concern, Ed," Wes said politely, "but I'll handle it."

"You can't meet them alone—" Wycoff said. Wes sensed a rising sense of indignation in Wycoff's voice.

Wanna make a bet? Wes thought. *The last thing I want is for employees to think I need you to protect me.* "That's my intent," Wes said pleasantly. "Involving members of the board in personnel problems will only complicate the issue. Let's set an early precedent, Mr. Wycoff—the employees deal with the administrator—not the board."

"Don't be a fool," Wycoff said spitting his words out with contempt. "A good CEO uses the talents of his board."

"Not in operations he doesn't."

Wycoff gasped at Wes's insolence. "As chairman of the Finance Committee, I plan to meet with our supervisors on the impending financial crisis," he said authoritatively.

Wes held his ground. "As chairman of the Finance Committee, you will meet only with the board. They will establish policy. I'll be the one to communicate that policy to the employees," he said. "I'm the hospital administrator, I'm responsible for operations."

Wycoff pushed on. "I must address a number of other issues with the employees. The budget, our new organizational structure."

This guy doesn't quit! "Those are operational issues," Wes repeated quietly but firmly. *Don't give in—we're setting precedent*, he thought.

Wycoff was silent. Wes could sense his anger. "Look, I appreciate your concern," Wes continued, "but if I need your help, I'll give you a call." Wes waved cheerfully at Dr. Flagg who stormed by without speaking.

"Good-bye, Wes," Wycoff said flatly.

Was that a parting salutation . . . or a threat? Wes wondered as he replaced the phone.

* * *

It took a heroic effort by housekeeping to arrange the cafeteria for a meeting with the employees on such short notice. The Dietary Department shut the breakfast line down promptly at 10:00 a.m.—thirty minutes early—as a team of housekeepers quickly descended on the department, removing tables, vacuuming, and setting up chairs.

Wes had one objective for the meeting—avert a walkout. The room filled quickly. He entered from the rear, making his way to a portable podium. "I'm Wes Douglas, your new administrator," he began. "I know many of you are surprised with my appointment—none of you more than I." *A feeble attempt at humor—no one smiled.*

Wes observed that the audience was divided into three groups. A small cluster standing in the back exchanged guffaws at their ringleader—a stocky maintenance man with a barrel chest and large animated arms that swung out from his body like hams as he mimicked Wes. From an earlier description, Wes assumed the comedian was Hank Ulman—the self-appointed union steward.

A second group, scattered throughout the audience, watched dispassionately, arms folded, faces skeptical, as though daring him to convince them the board hadn't made a mistake. The third group—ten or twelve people on the front row—appeared receptive. They were so small in number, however, that they were intimidated into silence by the others in the audience.

"I'd like to introduce myself by explaining my management philosophy," Wes continued. For the next ten minutes he discussed the goals he had established for the interim period of his administration, the most important of which was to put the hospital in the black.

"Now, talk to me about your concerns," he said after his brief presentation.

The room was momentarily silent. Then an employee from the Business Office raised her hand. "I have a complaint," she said. "The board never consults us, they don't even tell us what's going on. Not a single employee has ever heard of you, and suddenly you're the new boss." The room hummed with assent. "The newspaper editor knows more about what's going on around here than we do. Hap never told us about a financial crisis. How do we know it's real?"

"It's real," Wes replied.

"Can you guarantee there'll be no layoffs?" a nurse demanded.

"No. But your supervisors will be consulted before we reduce staff. There'll be no secrets."

A lab tech raised his hand. "The rumor is you're an accountant. I've got a complaint about Finance. The employees bear the brunt of revenue shortfalls, but it's not our fault—pricing is the problem. We're doing some of our lab tests for less than the cost of reagents."

"There's a bigger problem with waste," a nurse added. "On some units we throw away more sterile products than we use because of outdating."

Wes took notes. "Helpful input," he said. Complaints continued for another twenty minutes.

"There was a time in my career when I placed most of the problems of disorganization, poor quality, and service on the employees," Wes concluded.

36

"Experience has changed that perception. I've come to realize that the problem is often poor management. Give me a few days to find out what is going on," he said, "and we'll start hitting these issues straight on."

His approach seemed to be working. Many employees smiled—a few applauded. It was time to discuss the threatened walkout. As the morale of the meeting improved, he noticed Ulman's facial expressions grew more hostile. Suddenly Ulman left the room, taking with him two co-workers. *Good riddance,* Wes thought.

Wes was within striking distance of his objective, or so he thought. He cleared his throat. "There's one more issue I want to discuss," he said as the employees quieted. "Last evening an article in the paper reported a threatened employee walkout. The hospital has problems, but a walk-out won't solve them—"

A muffled explosion interrupted his words. It was followed by a loud hissing noise. A stream of boiling water, red with rust, gushed through the opening under the door leading to the boiler room and swirled over the feet of the employees. A female laundry worker in low cut shoes screamed in pain as she grabbed her ankles. A coworker grabbed her arm but slipped on the linoleum floor and fell in the scalding overflow. Two men pulled them from the water.

Ulman appeared in the doorway, interestingly enough, wearing hip boots. "A pipe to the boiler's broken!" he shouted. "Everyone out!"

The room exploded in commotion as the crowd convulsed to the front of the room, knocking over chairs in their efforts to escape the scalding flow. An employee hit the crash bar to the emergency exit, setting off the alarm as workers pushed one another through the door and up the stairwell. Ulman had successfully terminated the meeting.

✱ ✱ ✱

Thirty minutes later Wes called Ulman to his office.

"Like I tol' Hap, the boiler's old—needs replacin'." Ulman smiled, exposing a broken, chestnut-colored tooth. "Gonna kill somebody someday. The steam pipe came right off the wall. Good thing I was there. If I hadn't—well, things might have turned out differently."

"I'm sure that's true," Wes replied flatly.

A few minutes later, on his way out of the hospital, Wes checked in with Birdie. "Got a meeting at the bank," he said.

"I've scheduled the department heads for tomorrow," she replied. "Nine o'clock."

"Got it!" he replied, recording the appointment in his planner.

5

High Noon

Arnold Wilson stood angrily. Placing both hands on his desk, he leaned forward, thrusting his jaw threateningly in the face of young David Brannan. "Okay—I'll level with you, Dave. We've lost confidence in the hospital's ability to compete. Your controller can't even tell us where you're losing money!"

For twenty minutes, Wes Douglas had watched a jousting match. On the offensive was Arnold Wilson, vice president of Park City State Bank, scourging David Brannan for the hospital's poor financial performance. Wycoff, sitting in the corner, was uncharacteristically silent. Wes, the newcomer, said nothing. It was just as well—Wilson was doing his best to ignore him.

"Should've seen the reaction of the loan committee," throwing his hands up in disbelief, "when Selman told them the hospital doesn't even have accurate cost data on its products and procedures."

"Selman's your problem?" Brannan injected. "Selman's gone!"

"And who replaced him?" asked Wilson belligerently.

"We don't have a replacement," Brannan admitted.

"No controller? And a new administrator who's never worked in a hospital!" Wilson hooted. "No wonder the employees lost confidence in the board. Do you expect the directors of my bank to react differently?"

"I expect them to work with us until we resolve our problems," Brannan said evenly. "For thirty years we've been a good account—a loyal customer even when other banks were offering us lines of credit at much lower rates."

Wilson's brows lifted in an agonized expression. "David! We're not talking small amounts of money," he said. "By your own projections, you're looking at a fourth-quarter loss of $900,000."

Brannan was unimpressed. "If you call our line of credit, we won't be able to make payroll. Then our revenue stops—and we won't be able to pay you the money we owe you."

"You owe us $2 million," Wilson said, "collateralized by $3 million in accounts receivable." He snatched a thick file from his desk and thumbed to the third page. "Here it is—your total accounts receivable at the end of August was $3,078,000. We have an in-house collection agency; if the hospital closes, we'll collect the accounts ourselves. The worst option would be to sell the receivable outright." Wilson slapped the file closed. "A group in Ogden has agreed to buy your accounts for sixty cents on the dollar—that's a million eight in cash."

"It's $150,000 less than you'll get if you stick with us," Brannan countered.

"It's a million eight more than we have to lose if the hospital takes out bankruptcy," Wilson said. He shrugged. "Besides, that's the worst case scenario."

Wilson was interrupted as Hyrum Whittingham, president of the bank, stuck his head in the door. Whittingham had heard the bedlam and came down to see if he could help.

"Mind if I join you?"

Brannan motioned for him to enter. A muscle twitched nervously in Wilson's jaw. Face mottled, he popped a pill. Whittingham started to close the door, then noticed Wilson's agitation. He motioned for him to get a drink from the water cooler across the hall. Wilson left the room while Whittingham nodded at Wycoff, and then crossed the room to shake hands with David Brannan.

"How are you, David?" Whittingham asked, pumping his hand firmly.

"I've been better," David said, clipping his words. He gestured to Wes. "This is Wes Douglas—new administrator."

Whittingham shook hands with Wes and motioned for Brannan to sit down as he seated himself in Wilson's chair. Interlocking his fingers, he leaned forward. "What seems to be the problem?" he asked with a frigid smile.

Brannan's eyes blazed—hot enough, Wes thought, to ignite the paneling on the wall. "You know very well what's the problem!" Brannan barked angrily. "The bank's canceled our line of credit. Without it, we can't meet payroll. I want to know who's responsible!"

Wilson reentered the office, and Whittingham motioned for him to shut the door. By now, Brannan's shouting was attracting the attention of customers in the lobby.

Whittingham arched his eyebrows. "I'm responsible," he said. "Some people think the money we loan out is our own—they think they're borrowing the funds of a group of wealthy investors who own the bank. That's not the case, David."

Whittingham made no attempt to hide the sarcasm in his voice. "The money we loan comes from depositors—school teachers saving for retirement, young couples planning for a home, small merchants trying to scratch out a living . . . we have a responsibility to those people, David. A responsibility to see that those funds are wisely invested—that they aren't squandered on organizations that can't manage their own finances."

"Don't give me that trash!" Brannan spat the words out contemptuously. "For twenty years, my father was a major shareholder in this bank. I know what banking's about."

Whittingham nodded, his face flushing with anger. "Your father's not a shareholder anymore," he said, his words short and biting. He picked up a copy of the bank's annual report and shook it in the air. "This committee calls the shots now," he said, slapping the picture of the new directors on the cover. He slammed the report down on the table. "We have a new loan committee, David. Would you like to know the committee's criteria for new and existing loans?"

Before David could reply, Whittingham continued, his words coming out in staccato-like burst. "Loans must be *collateralized,*" he said with scouring emphasis. "Loans can't exceed 70 percent *of collateral.* Borrowers must have *positive cash flows.* Borrowers must demonstrate their ability to *pay their loans back!"*

"Why, David," Whittingham continued sarcastically, "your hospital doesn't meet a single criterion. We have *no choice* but to call the loan!"

The room was quiet as Brannan digested Whittingham's message. Wes was not aware David's father had been an owner in the bank. His withdrawal—for whatever reason—had obviously precipitated a shift in power that Brannan was just beginning to comprehend.

From the corner, Wycoff appeared to be enjoying the whipping Brannan was taking. Sitting next to him, Wilson, arms folded, stared at Whittingham approvingly. Brannan glanced at Wycoff, who gave no support, and then glared at Whittingham. Everyone expected Wycoff to speak, but he said nothing.

Sensing the meeting was about to end with disastrous results for the hospital, Wes interjected himself into the conversation for the first time. "I understand your commitment to your shareholders and to your depositors," he said calmly. "That's why I find it hard to believe you're willing to see the community's only hospital go out of business."

"There are other hospitals in the area," Whittingham said defensively. "Some firm just built a new one in Midway—eleven miles from here. It's not too far to go for healthcare."

"I'm not talking healthcare, I'm talking economics," Wes said, taking the offensive. "Peter Brannan Community Hospital has about two hundred employees. Surely you don't believe it's to the benefit of your depositors for the community to lose its largest employer."

A question shadowed Whittingham's eyes. "What do you mean?" he asked.

Wycoff smiled and shifted forward, taking an interest in the conversation for the first time. Wilson swallowed another pill.

"The hospital spends $12 million a year on payroll. I have data showing that sixty-five percent of the payroll dollars are spent locally. Every dollar of payroll generates an additional dollar in secondary spending within the community. In total, the hospital is responsible for $16 million a year in local spending." Wes paused for effect. "Are your directors willing to take that money from their depositors?"

Whittingham looked annoyed. "Who said anything about taking money from our depositors?"

"Who gets the $16 million?" Wes asked. "Your customers, the local merchants. Many of those merchants have loans with your bank. With that reduction in income, how many will be able to service those loans?"

"Most of our employees are customers of the bank," Wes continued. "If the hospital closes, many will be forced to leave the community to find employment. As they leave, so will their deposits. Most of these people own homes—mortgaged by your bank. As one or two hundred homes hit the market, what will happen to the price of real estate in the community? What will be the effect on the bank as real estate values fall and your collateral in these homes dries up?"

The room was silent as Whittingham digested Wes's message. He bounced a questioning look off Wilson. "Is that the hospital's loan file?" he asked, pointing to the folder on Wilson's desk.

"It is," Wilson replied.

"Bring it with you. Let's meet in my office." Whittingham stood to leave and then turned to Wes. "Give us a few minutes—we'll see what we can do."

* * *

"Gentlemen, we have a proposition for you," Wilson said, when he and Whittingham returned. Whittingham had delegated the meeting back to Wilson, who took a seat at his desk. Whittingham stood, arms folded, at the door.

"We'll continue to work with the hospital for ninety days, at the end of which time we'll reevaluate our financial relationship," Wilson announced. "Our conditions are as follows: Within thirty days you'll provide a business plan showing how you'll compete profitably in your new fixed-price environment. Within 90 days you'll be at breakeven. Within 120 days, you will consistently achieve an operating margin of at least 3 percent of gross revenue. We assume you won't be able to reach that without layoffs and a restructuring of your entire operation," he concluded, looking up from the notes he had taken in Whittingham's office.

"The accounting system . . . you forgot the cost accounting system," interrupted Whittingham.

"Oh, yes. Within sixty days, you must have a cost accounting system in place that can accurately report product cost. We anticipate these costs will be reflected in your updated business plan."

"I think we can do that," Wes said.

Wilson paused for a moment to look at Whittingham, who nodded for him to continue. "There's one last requirement," Wilson added. "Unless you're willing to meet this final requirement, the deal's off. We're asking for a security interest on your equipment, including your new MRI unit. We also want to hold the title to the land you purchased north of town for the new hospital."

Brannan sat up. "That's a little stiff," he complained. "The MRI was purchased with a grant from the Mike and Sara Brannan Foundation. We were hoping to hold the land unencumbered—even if we can't build a new hospital at this time, there's a partially finished doctors' office building on the property."

"Those are our requirements," Wilson stated with finality.

Edward Wycoff, who had been taking notes, looked up. "I have an alternative suggestion," he said, choosing his words carefully. "I don't know how the Brannan family will feel about a lien on the MRI the foundation gave the hospital. They've made a significant contribution over the years—it would be a shame to turn our backs on that support."

David Brannan gave Wycoff a look of disbelief mixed with gratitude—it was the first time David could remember that Wycoff had spoken favorably of the Brannan family.

Wycoff continued, addressing Whittingham directly. "Your last requirement closes the door on a number of options our interim administrator might need in order to turn the hospital around. I think there's a better way."

"I'm listening," Whittingham said cautiously.

"What if I were willing to guarantee the line of credit up to $2 million? The bank would still have the loan—collateralized of course by the accounts receivable. All the requirements you stipulated would remain in effect *except the security interest in the equipment, and the lien on the property.*"

41

"I think the loan committee might approve something like that," Whittingham responded. "What do you think, David?"

"I think it's a gracious offer," Brannan responded. "I'll have the hospital's attorney draw the note up."

"My attorney insists on doing that," Wycoff interrupted.

"What?" Brannan asked.

"The note would be guaranteed by stock I've set up in a family trust. My attorney, who also serves as trustee of my estate, is a fairly astute businessman. I've discussed it with him, and he has stipulated that the trust must receive the first liens.

"The trust, of course, doesn't want to own an MRI or 100 acres of land," Wycoff said assuringly. "But an arrangement of this kind would serve as an incentive for management to take the actions necessary to put Peter Brannan Community Hospital in the black."

Brannan was silent. The gratitude had vanished from his eyes. Wycoff was the smarter of the two, and he knew it. His father had never trusted Wycoff. Still, David Brannan was unable to guarantee the note himself; and for his family's sake, he didn't want to see the hospital close. He pondered the situation momentarily and then nodded his assent.

Whittingham grinned broadly. "Good! I'll arrange for the bank's attorney to meet with your trustee," he said, holding his hand out to Wycoff. "Hopefully we've happened on an agreement that will assure the hospital's continued operation while protecting the bank."

"I'm sure it will be to our common benefit," Wycoff replied.

* * *

Although the weatherman had forecast rain, the sun was shining through scattered clouds as Wes left the bank, grateful for the help offered by Edward Wycoff. *I misjudged Wycoff,* he thought. *Few board members would be willing to risk their own money to save a community hospital. There's more at stake than I thought. This is a great guy—I mustn't let him down.*

* * *

Alone in the bank's conference room, Wycoff placed a long-distance call. "Mr. Devecchi, please," he said when a secretary answered. She put the call through immediately.

"Devecchi," he said. "This is Wycoff—they bought it! Yeah, I gave Wes Douglas just enough rope to hang himself. No, I don't think Brannan suspects anything. Yes, we've got the liens, they have ninety days . . . and then we've got 'em."

6

Never Give Up

Wes often thought about his grandfather, Admiral Wesley E. Douglas, a naval engineer with degrees from Annapolis, the Massachusetts Institute of Technology, and Harvard Business School. Grandfather Douglas was a man of detail, discipline, and accomplishment. In subtle ways Wes was just beginning to understand, grandfather had significantly shaped his value system.

In the 1970s, Grandfather Douglas had encouraged Wes to join a local troop of the Boy Scouts. He realized that fourteen year-old Wes needed a better outlet for adolescent energies than girls and skateboarding.

Wes quickly climbed from the rank of Tenderfoot to Life Scout. At sixteen he was ready to tackle the rank of Eagle. One requirement is the eagle project, typically a constructive activity of significant magnitude to teach the principles of self-reliance, determination, and service. Concerned with the environment, Wes had chosen the restoration of a nature trail in one of Maine's state parks. Wes had proposed clearing a five-mile trail, with the construction of park benches every quarter mile, and a small pavilion at the three-mile mark.

Grandfather Douglas, an engineer by training, reviewed Wes's proposal and warned him that the project might be too large for a boy of his age. Wes knew better, or so he thought, and the proposal was submitted as written. In later years, Wes would learn to take counsel from those older and wiser.

Wes started his project June 1st, as soon as school concluded. His plan was to finish by the first of July. By the middle of July, he reached the half way mark. The park ranger was a stickler for detail, with a vision that exceeded Wes's. It was just too much work. While Wes's friends spent their summer swimming, chasing girls or earning money for clothes, he cleared weeds, hauled rocks, built benches and painted outhouses. By August 1st he was ready to give up.

He talked with his dad who encouraged him to see the project through to completion. Certain that he would find an ally in his grandfather, who had discouraged him from proposing such a large project in the first place, Wes bicycled that evening to Grandfather Douglas's home.

His grandfather listened patiently while Wes explained how difficult the project had become, and how foolish it would be to waste the remaining summer completing it. Wes' grandfather listened patiently, never interrupting. When the boy had finished, he spoke.

"You made a commitment that's going to be difficult to fulfill," Grandfather said sympathetically. "But, before you renege, you need to think about the consequences."

"Consequences?" young Wes asked.

"Consequences," grandfather affirmed. "As unhappy as you are with the park ranger, he spent considerable time planning and supervising the project. He also went to bat for you, persuading the Parks Department to purchase the lumber for the benches and pavilion. You made a commitment, and others donated resources based on that commitment."

Wes could see where the conversation was headed—he didn't like it. "What the ranger wants me to do isn't reasonable," he protested.

"Maybe, but you participated in the design, and you signed the contract."

"But Grandfather, it's ruining my summer!"

Grandfather nodded. "Better your summer than your reputation."

"I don't care what others think."

"I do," he said. "You share my name."

Young Wes was silent, shamed by the truthfulness of his grandfather's logic.

"A reputation is an important thing," grandfather continued. "It's not just your reputation that I'm concerned about, however, it's your character. Character is formed by habits, and habits are formed by actions. This isn't the first time you'll face a task that's bigger than you are. Quit now and you'll set a precedent, establish a habit. The next time you face opposition it will be all that much easier to retreat. Reinforce the habit, and you'll eventually loose the strength to succeed."

For the remainder of the summer, Wes's grandfather drove him each day to the state park, where they both completed the project just before school began. It was one of the most meaningful experiences of young Wes's life. Wes learned what it means to persevere in the face of immense obstacles. It wasn't just an Eagle Project that Grandfather Douglas molded that summer, it was a grandson.

Twelve years after the death of his grandfather, Wes revisited the park. With permission from the State Park Service, he placed a small plaque where the trail ended. On it was a quote by Winston Churchill—a quote his grandfather had repeated numerous times that summer.

"Never give up," Churchill said, *"Never, never, never give up!"*

* * *

That afternoon Wes met with the hospital's supervisors to formulate a plan to put the hospital at breakeven within ninety days.

"What obstacles do you face in running your departments?" he asked as the meeting began.

Jeff Lee, director of the laboratory, spoke first. "Most problems relate to our losses. For many years, the hospital was profitable. Some departments made money on less volume than they're running now. I've heard that the problem is *Managed Care*. I don't know what that means. Wycoff tells us healthcare operates in a new environment and we have to manage differently, but no one ever tells us how."

Wes wrote on the board:

Managed care—training and management

"I don't know much about managed care either," said June Hammer, the chief dietitian, "except Cluff told me that it involves something called *prospective payment*. He said we get paid less under this payment system, although I've never seen a report to verify that's true—as a matter of fact I rarely see any type of accounting report."

Wes wrote:

Prospective payment
Possible losses
Accounting reports

Elizabeth Flannigan, Director of Nursing, spoke next. A scrappy Irish woman with flaming red hair, Elizabeth was famous for her skirmishes with the medical staff. She was not the type to take guff from anybody. "Our budgeting system stinks," she said bluntly. "The forms we're asked to fill out each year are impossible to understand, and there's no one to answer questions."

Barry Lindeman, the laundry manager, agreed. "Some of us spend a lot of time preparing forecasts and budgets. When they come back, cuts have been made without our input or consent. It's stupid to hold us accountable for budgets we didn't prepare," he said, his face flushing red.

"This isn't a recent phenomenon," Elizabeth added. The controller's office has never been responsive to our needs. They think we work for them—I always thought it was supposed to be the other way around." Wes nodded, writing on the board:

Poor budgeting system
Unresponsive controller's office

"Most of the time we can't understand what they're talkin' about," Barrry chimed in. "They use fancy terms like *amortization* and *lee-quidity*. They have their own language—they do. Why . . . they're harder to understand than the Docs."

Elizabeth nodded in approval. "We don't get reports that are useful for decision making," she said. "In addition, the reports aren't fair. We're judged by our bottom line—but many departments have indirect costs allocated against them. We don't control indirect costs."

"Financial reports aren't timely," complained June Hammer. "What good are January's reports in May?"

Turning to the board, Wes wrote:

No service orientation
Poor communication
Reports—unacceptable format and untimely

"Other problems?" Wes inquired.

The room was silent. "Those are the major ones," Elizabeth said finally. "Give us the tools we need to run our departments and we'll fix our own problems."

"You'll get 'em," Wes replied.

7

A Dynasty Falls

Perched high on a hill overlooking the small resort town of Park City is the Brannan Mansion. Constructed in 1896 in a Victoria Gothic style, its high Venetian tower reflects the arrogance and energy of its builder, Mike Brannan—an Irishman who struck it rich in the silver mines of Park City in the late 1880s.

Ornate wrought-iron doors, added more for decoration than protection—guard an outdoor vestibule. Beyond those gates stand large double doors of carved oak and beveled glass; beyond those doors lie waterfall staircases and paneled nooks, warmly lit by stained glass.

Deep within the bowels of the mansion is the library. Roughly thirty feet square, the room is interlaced with loggias and balconies, its formal design contrasting sharply with the Gothic asymmetry of the other rooms of the nineteenth-century mansion.

David Brannan hadn't been in this room since he left for college—he preferred his condominium above the Stein Erickson ski lodge overlooking Park City. Today, however, he had come to sign documents that would dissolve a financial empire built by three generations of the Brannan family.

It was 3:30 in the afternoon, and David poured himself another drink. Replacing the bottle on the heavily carved walnut desk his great-grandfather had imported from Italy, he toasted a portrait of the old goat that hung high above the hand-carved marble fireplace.

Michael James Brannan had immigrated to the United States in 1882 from Monahan, Ireland. Arriving through the Port of New York, he and his brother Patrick remained long enough to visit family and buy supplies before heading west for the gold fields of California. They never reached their destination. Stopping in Salt Lake City for supplies, Mike fell in love with a Mormon girl, married, and never left Utah.

For a while, Mike and his brother tried farming. They failed miserably. Mike wasn't a Mormon, and he wasn't a farmer. Rumors of the discovery of silver on a spur not far from Dayton Peak soon drew him to the ledges and peaks of the Rocky Mountains east of Salt Lake City.

The American Lode was the first mining claim in the district. It was not until the discovery of the Ontario mine in 1879, however, that Park City began to flourish. Purchased in 1872 by George Hearst, father of William Randolph Hearst, the Ontario Mine would produce $50 million in silver ore. Later mines—the Pinion, the Walker, the Webster, the Flagstaff, the McHenry and the Buckeye—would produce a dozen or so family fortunes, including that of the Brannans.

As David studied the portrait, his eyes shimmered with genuine curiosity. He wondered what the old boy would think if he could see the family today. Gone were the silver and coal mines, the bank, the newspaper, and the hotel. All that was left was the stock in a small software firm that would provide enough money to fund a small trust for David's mother. He took another drink, wiping his mouth with the back of his hand, and set the tumbler back on the table.

Part of the family's financial disaster might have been avoided if his father, James Brannan, had not insisted in running the business late into his eighties. Much of the family income came from coal mines in Carbon County—the silver mines had long ago been closed.

David's father resisted modernization, pumping money into highly speculative ventures, including a software company. These required huge amounts of cash, jeopardizing the family's liquidity. Facing the possible loss of his investment, he flipped 180 degrees, spending $6 million on improvements and mining equipment. The market for coal was depressed, however. Strapped for cash, Brannan Inc. collapsed like a house of cards. Unable to cope with failure, James suffered a massive stroke in February, dying early in March. David Brannan inherited the family business, along with some of the blame for its collapse.

David's eyes flashed with anger as he studied the photograph of his father on the desk. With a violent sweep of his arm, he knocked it off, the glass shattering as the sterling-silver frame smashed into the stone mantle of the ornate fireplace and bounced onto the marble floor. He studied it for a moment—broken at his feet—and then poured another drink.

David was not like his father—or his father's father, or his father before him. He hated the family business as much as he hated his father. Given a choice, he would have opted for a professorship in history or literature at some small Ivy League college.

He wasn't given a choice, however. Free agency wasn't a part of the Brannan family vocabulary—not where children were concerned. Jim enrolled his son in engineering at the Colorado School of Mines with the idea that one day David would take over the family's operations. David took two quarters of math and flunked out of school. Later, with financial help from his mother, he completed a degree in American Studies from a small college in the East. He taught at a small college in Minnesota before returning home to settle his father's estate.

David was grateful to his mother—she had been the only buffer between him and the unpredictable wrath of his father. For his mother's sake, he had done his best to save what remained of the family's fortune. There wasn't much left to save, however, and he didn't know how to save it anyway.

His thoughts were interrupted by voices in the parlor. His mother hosted the Ladies Auxiliary of the hospital the last Wednesday of every month. She was not fully aware of the family situation. Her home was unencumbered, and David hoped to obtain enough money from the sale of the remaining businesses to maintain her in a reasonable manner for the rest of her life. At eighty-two years of age, she deserved better than this.

David's shoulders rose and fell as he sighed deeply. Studying the documents on the desk, he slowly picked up a pen and signed the declaration of bankruptcy. The hospital wasn't the only organization in the community with financial difficulties.

8

Why Are Costs So High?

The first snow of the season was blanketing the foothills as a blue Taurus broke out of Parley's Canyon east of Salt Lake City on Interstate 80. Wes Douglas caught a glimpse of the valley. He had first visited Salt Lake City with his parents in the 1970s. It was surprising the changes that had taken place since then.

In the distance, a cluster of skyscrapers, majestic and tall, like the lofty mountains, all but encompassed the granite towers of the Mormon Temple—a landmark that for so many years dominated the skyline. To the north, high on a hill, the State Capitol Building stood herald over the valley, its copper dome reflecting a history of mining and mineral exploration—an important counterpoint to the ecclesiastical history of the state. Originally settled by Mormon pioneers in 1847, later joined by prospectors and soldiers, and home of the 2002 Winter Olympics, the state had become as diverse as its scenery.

The purpose of Wes's trip was to meet with the hospital's auditors in Salt Lake City. With a ninety-day mandate from the bank to reach breakeven, he needed to understand more about hospital accounting and finance. The CPA firm that prepared the hospital's financial statements was a good place to start. Wes took the Sixth South Street exit downtown. Parking in the basement of the Utah One Building, he caught an elevator to the tenth floor where he announced himself to the accounting firm's receptionist, then took a seat.

In less than a minute, Karisa Holyoak, managing partner, appeared. She was tall and slender and had a bewitching smile that faintly reminded him of Kathryn. Her eyes sparkled with enthusiasm and intelligence.

Karisa led him to a small conference room. "This is your first week on the job," she said, taking a seat directly across from Wes at the conference table. She looked at him with wide and curious eyes. "Usually it takes me longer than that to get in trouble with a new client. How can I help you?"

"I think I'm the one in trouble," Wes murmured, mirroring her expression. "I'm trying to understand how a hospital that charges $1,800 a day can run at a loss."

Karisa smiled—she'd considered the question. "Our firm's had the hospital account for twenty years," she informed him. She opened the hospital's audit file and laid it on the table. "For many years, the hospital was one of our most stable clients."

Karisa thumbed through several reports, opening the most recent audit. "About three years ago, the hospital's financial position started a downward spiral," she continued, reading from her notes. Although volume went up, revenue went down. We concluded that the problem was managed care."

"What's that?" Wes inquired.

"It's an insurer approach to cost control. It's having an effect on the way hospitals manage their business. Peter Brannan Community Hospital seems to be having more difficulty with it than others. We tried to do an analysis to determine what products were losing money, but the hospital doesn't have a cost accounting system. The data needed for the analysis simply isn't available."

Wes nodded in agreement. "I need better data to run the hospital. I feel like a pilot flying without instruments."

"Good analogy," replied Karisa. "You're not only flying in the dark, but you're running out of fuel. Unless things change, we project you will be out of cash in another two to three months."

Wes sighed. "It might not take that long. Any suggestions on how I should proceed?"

Raising her eyebrows, Karisa leaned forward. "May I be candid?" she asked.

"Please," Wes nodded.

"You seem like a nice guy, Wes, but you're out of your league. I know you're a CPA, but you don't know the first thing about hospitals. By the time you learn the rules, the game'll be over."

Wes agreed. Five days on the job had convinced him that managing a hospital was different from anything he had previously experienced. The assumptions were different, even the terminology was new. The departments in the hospital were like separate countries—each with its own customs and language.

"What do you suggest?" he asked.

"Find another job . . . or find a mentor."

"I can't quit," he said. "There's too much at stake."

"For you or the hospital?"

"Both."

Karisa nodded knowingly.

"Can you suggest a mentor?" he asked.

"I don't know anyone who has all the answers, but I can put you in contact with someone who might get you started. We occasionally use the services of a health economist at the University Hospital—a fellow by the name of Herb Krimmel," Karisa said, retrieving his address from her computer. "Dr. Krimmel has an interesting background—he's a physician with a degree in health economics. He teaches at the University Hospital. Coincidentally, he lives in Park City."

Opening her day planner, Karisa wrote a note. "Let me give him a call," she said. "I think he'll be willing to talk to you. You might ask him to introduce you to the University Hospital's controller. University Hospital has an impressive cost accounting system in place. Maybe you can borrow some of their ideas."

Karisa gave him a dazzling smile, stood, and held out her hand. "Hope I've been helpful," she said.

Wes took her hand and shook it warmly. "Thanks. I'll be in touch."

* * *

Thursday evening, Wes received a phone call from Karisa telling him she had spoken with Krimmel. "As it works out, his car's in for service," she said. "Since he's a neighbor, he wondered if he could catch a ride to University Hospital with you tomorrow morning. He promised to set you up with the people who can explain what's happening in the industry." She paused. "You'll find him a little eccentric, but I think you'll like him."

After hanging up, Wes called Krimmel, and made arrangements to pick him up at his home the next morning.

9

A Lesson in Medical Economics

Krimmel's home, a two-story farmhouse, was three miles north of Park City. The doctor was waiting for him at the curb. "I'm Herb Krimmel," he said as he opened the car door. Climbing in, he brushed the residue of what looked like cornmeal from his tweed coat and trousers onto the floor. "Breakfast is always a mess."

Wes looked at him oddly. "Yours?"

"No, the chickens!" Krimmel replied. "Run a small farm. The wife would like me to sell 'em, but I wake up early—old age you know, and it gives me something to do before she gets up." His eyes twinkled. "Besides, the chickens are the only ones around here who listen to me."

Krimmel laughed. Wes couldn't help but laugh too as he studied his odd traveling companion. Short and chubby, Krimmel had curly red hair, a large Roman nose, and round horn-rimmed glasses that looked like small fishbowls, as they magnified his eyes in a peculiar sort of way. Wes turned onto the highway.

"You're new on the job?"

"Fifth day."

"And no experience?"

"Not in hospitals."

Krimmel raised one eyebrow "You've chosen an interesting time to enter the field. How's it going?"

Wes's nodded his head up and down, then left to right as though he couldn't agree with himself. "Good . . . actually, not so good," he confessed.

Smiling, Krimmel was silent as he studied the cornmeal at his feet. "Ought to vacuum your car more often," he said.

"I'm told that our medical director's an old friend of yours." Wes said.

"Whose that?" Krimmel asked.

"Dr. Emil Flagg."

Krimmel chuckled. "An old friend? Wouldn't go that far. We were classmates in medical school. Both courted the same girl, I won of course." He arched his eyebrows mischievously. "Always felt he was a bad sport," Krimmel said with a grin. "How do you get along with him?"

"Don't know—only talked with him once. Didn't go that well, it was more a confrontation than a meeting. Flagg thinks medicine's too commercial—thinks there's too much emphasis on the bottom line. Blames businessmen like Edward Wycoff, for the trend."

"Who's Wycoff?"

"Our Finance Committee Chairman, a retired investment banker. He thinks I'm his ally."

"Are you?" Krimmel asked.

"Not sure," Wes looked quizzically at Krimmel. "That's part of the reason I came to see you."

"Emil and I were in the same class in medical school—the class of 1964," Krimmel said. "It was a different era—stressed quality, paid little attention to cost. One reason was that costs were low. When Emil and I graduated the room rate at the University Hospital was $40 a day—total costs including x-ray, lab, and pharmacy were about $80."

"What are they today?"

"Twenty-five hundred bucks."

Wes whistled softly. "That's a lot of money," he said. "Why are they so high?"

"Technology. Construction costs for new hospitals can exceed $250,000 per bed, including the investment in medical equipment."

"Is there anything hospital administrators can do?"

"They can be careful not to overbuild," Krimmel replied. "Duplication's expensive. When I was a medical student at the University of Colorado Medical School in Denver, there were twenty-two hospitals in town. All of them were operating at 60 percent occupancy, and most of them had expensive construction projects underway to expand their capacity."

"Why build, if you aren't at full capacity?" Wes asked.

"Several reasons," Krimmel replied. "Prestige, salary, a desire to provide the medical staff with the latest technology, and job security. Physicians and patients alike seemed to share the *"bigger-is-better"* syndrome. Patients equate size with quality."

"What's size have to do with salary?" Wes asked.

"Hospital administrators' salaries typically correlate with number of beds. The greater the number of beds, the larger the paycheck."

"What about job security?"

"It's difficult to fire an administrator in the middle of a building project," Krimmel replied. "A three-year building project provides three years of additional security for an administrator in trouble with the board."

"You sound cynical," Wes said.

"A little. In all fairness, that's probably the least important reason, however. The biggest issue is technology."

"Isn't technology good?"

"Yeah, but it has to be used efficiently."

"Can't hospitals share equipment?" Wes asked.

"After graduating from medical school, I did my residency at St. Joseph's Hospital in Chicago—a fine facility. While I was there, Presbyterian Hospital directly across the street installed a million-dollar piece of equipment for use in their cancer treatment program. Shortly thereafter, the board at St. Joseph's announced they planned to build a similar facility."

Krimmel shook his head in disbelief as he recalled the experience. "One afternoon, while the residents were doing rounds, we confronted our administrator in the hall. One of my classmates asked her if she had considered the effect this would have on the community's total healthcare cost—Presbyterian's facility was only being utilized at 30 percent of capacity," Krimmel added.

"'Why not share Presbyterian's facility?' he asked. I'll never forget her answer!"
"'Young man,' she said, 'when it comes to patient care, cost is not an issue. At St. Joseph's we don't compete on the basis of cost, we compete on the basis of quality!'"

Krimmel swore under his breath. "It was a bunch of bull, of course. The real reason St. Joseph's was unwilling to use Presbyterian's equipment had nothing to do with quality—Presbyterian's cancer center had a national reputation. But Presbyterian Hospital was St. Joseph's main competitor. The administrator opposed anything that would send her doctors to a competing facility, even if it drove patient cost up."

"One of the problems," Krimmel continued is the health care industry lacks some incentives that promote cost control through price competition."

"Why didn't hospitals compete on the basis of cost?" Wes asked. "Other industries are price competitive."

"Do you know much about economics?"

"I had a class in graduate school, it wasn't my favorite subject," Wes admitted.

Krimmel nodded. "Before I decided to go to medical school, I majored in economics. I teach a medical economics course to fourth-year medical students."

"Karisa mentioned that," said Wes.

"One of the characteristics for price competition is a free market," Krimmel continued. "Do you remember the conditions necessary for a free market to exist?"

"I think so—" Wes said thoughtfully. "A free market requires a consumer who makes the decision to purchase, shops on the basis of quality and price, and negotiates an arms-length purchase price."

Impressed, Krimmel raised his eyebrows. "That's good," he said. "I'll have to invite you to speak to my class."

Wes looked at Dr. Krimmel warily but said nothing.

"Let's talk about how the market mechanism works in most industries. Then let's compare that with what happens in the healthcare industry."

From the animated expression on Krimmel's face, it was apparent he enjoyed this topic. Despite a couple of kinks in his personality, Wes suspected he was a good teacher.

"You're driving a new car," Krimmel said.

"A new Taurus," Wes corrected.

"Fine . . . let's talk about the market mechanism in the auto industry. Who decided you needed a new car?"

"I did."

"Why did you think you needed a new car?" Krimmel pressed.

"The second transmission fell out of my Yugo."

"All right, you were a consumer who could assess his needs for transportation."

"That's right," Wes said, "I met the first requirement for a free market."

"What did you tell me was the second?"

"The consumer must shop on the basis of quality and price," Wes answered.

"Did you do that?" Krimmel asked.

"Yes."

"How?"

"I read the automobile reviews in *Consumer Reports*. I also talked to people who owned models I was interested in."

"Was price a consideration?"

"Yes."

"Did you negotiate?"

"Yes."

"How?"

"By visiting competing dealers and bargaining with the salesmen."

"You're sure price was important to you?"

"Absolutely," Wes said.

"If the price had been too high, you wouldn't have bought a Taurus?"

"Probably not."

"What if price dropped, let's say by 50 percent?"

"Well," Wes replied, " might have bought two vehicles—one for work and one for the mountains."

"Do you remember what economists call a change in demand caused by a change in price?"

"Price elasticity," Wes said with emphasis. He remembered something about economics after all.

"Wes—you're good!" Dr. Krimmel said in mock amazement. "Automobile manufacturers and dealers have incentives to keep their prices as low as possible, consistent with quality, since they compete on the basis of quality and price. It looks like the market mechanism works for the automobile industry."

Wes was satisfied with the explanation. "I'll buy that," he said.

"Now let's talk about the traditional healthcare industry. Assume you wake up one morning with a pain in your belly. You palpate your abdomen, run a few tests and decide you need a cholecystectomy—right?"

"Wrong . . . I don't know anything about medicine. What's a cholecystectomy, anyway?" Wes asked.

"An operation to remove a gall bladder." Krimmel studied Wes thoughtfully. "So who decides if you'll purchase a lab test or an operation?"

"My doctor."

"And who provides the product?"

"My doctor."

"Who prices the product?"

"My doctor."

"You're repeating yourself . . ."

"I noticed," Wes said.

"Why delegate all that to your doctor?" Krimmel asked skeptically.

"He understands medicine—I don't."

"That's our first problem," Krimmel replied. "Economists call it unequal, or *disparate,* information."

Wes was silent, then nodded. Krimmel continued. "Do you think disparate information's a greater problem in medicine than it is in say the automobile industry?"

"Probably."

"What if society were organized in such a way that it was the auto salesmen who decided when and if their customers bought new cars?"

"It would be a nice world for auto dealers, but I'm not sure how good it would be for the consumer."

"Why?"

"Salesmen make money by selling products. They'd have an incentive to sell products the customer might not need."

"Maybe that's the situation in healthcare," Krimmel said.

Wes' eyes widened with recognition as he understood for the first time the economic power of the physician.

"Okay," Krimmel continued, "we've determined that the healthcare industry fails the first test of a free market—the consumer doesn't make the decision to purchase. Once the decision to buy has been made, does the consumer shop on the basis of quality and price?"

"Consumers have a difficult time judging quality in healthcare," Wes said.

"Why?"

"Disparate information," Wes replied mouthing the new term.

"That's right," Krimmel noted. "Studies indicate that patients judge the quality of hospital care by its *hotel services*—the cleanliness of the room, the friendliness of the personnel, the quality of the food. You probably don't shop on the basis of price either, do you?" Dr. Krimmel asked.

"Probably not."

"At least *I've* never had a patient ask *me* where he could get a cheap cholecystectomy," Krimmel said. "Do you know why?" he continued.

"Prices aren't available."

"Any other reasons?"

"People equate low price with lack of quality. No one wants a shoddy operation."

"And . . . ?" Krimmel prodded.

Wes grinned. "Who wants to drive a hard bargain with a doctor whose going to cut you open tomorrow."

Krimmel laughed. "I never thought about that," he remarked slapping himself on the knee. "Very good! Seriously though, let's talk about price elasticity. If you were perfectly healthy and the surgeon ran a special on cholecystectomies—a complete operation for $1,225—how many would you buy?"

"None."

"What if the price were lowered to $200?" Krimmel inquired.

"If I were healthy, I wouldn't buy one," Wes responded.

"What if your daughter had a brain tumor, and the cost of the life-saving surgery was $125. How many brain operations would you buy?"

"One, of course."

"What if the price was $10,000?"

"I would still just buy one operation."

"A million dollars?"

"For my little girl—I'd try to find a way."

"Ha!" said Krimmel. "So price *doesn't* influence the quantity of healthcare goods and services purchased—there's little or no price elasticity."

"For many products, that's probably true," Wes responded grimly.

Krimmel was silent as he collected his thoughts. "When consumers fail to shop on the basis of price, incentives for cost control by suppliers tend to disappear," he said. "That's another reason healthcare costs are so high."

"While we are on the subject of cost incentives," Dr. Krimmel continued, "there's one other factor in the equation I should mention. Traditionally, most patients didn't select their hospital—their physician also made that decision. Consequently, many hospitals viewed the physician and not the patient as their primary customer."

"How did that increase cost?" Wes asked.

"Let me give you an example," Krimmel explained. "When I was doing my residency at St. Joseph's Hospital, I moonlighted in the emergency center at Presbyterian. One day, Presbyterian hired a new administrator, a person who felt she needed to do something to reduce the cost of healthcare.

"Since physicians control approximately 70 percent of the cost of the average hospital," Krimmel continued, "she decided to focus on the medical staff first. The first thing she did was to tell the physicians they were no longer going to purchase excess medical equipment. If one group of physicians wanted Sony heart monitors for surgery and another wanted Sylvania, the two groups would have to get together and agree on one brand. They would no longer duplicate equipment just to keep people happy. The hospital also looked at the 'freebies' the doctors were getting—free meals in the cafeteria, free laundry, free treatment and drug prescriptions for family illnesses, etc. Cost control was the new administrator's focus.

"St. Joseph's hospital administrator took a different approach," Krimmel continued. "He told me it was his philosophy to keep the medical staff happy. *Give the physicians what they want*, was his motto."

Dr. Krimmel gave Wes a searching look. "Guess who wound up with most of the patients—the hospital that tried to control cost or the hospital that courted its medical staff?" Dr. Krimmel asked.

"Probably the hospital that gave the doctors what they wanted."

"Why?"

"Because it was the doctor and not the patient who selected the hospital."

Krimmel gave him a thumbs-up. "You've got it," he crowed. "A study conducted in 1975 showed that many hospitals were operated in a manner to maximize the income of their physicians," Krimmel continued. "One way to do that was to provide excess capacity. Under fee-for-service, a physician's income is a function of the time he or she spends treating patients. Physicians waiting in line to access hospital equipment or facilities are not seeing patients—or earning money."

Krimmel looked directly at Wes. "When I first joined the staff of University Hospital, most of our surgeons were screaming for additional operating rooms. Operating rooms are expensive to build. The administrator looked at the surgical schedule and found that the operating rooms were being used only 60 percent of the time.

"He couldn't understand the physician's demands. What he failed to realize, however, was that despite the low utilization, there were still times when more than one physician needed the same operating suite. When an emergency arose, someone was bumped from the schedule or had to wait to get into surgery. Downtime is costly from the standpoint of the physician."

"Then the ideal world from a physician's standpoint would be to have one operating room, completely staffed and equipped and on-call at all times, for every surgeon?" Wes asked.

"Yes, as long as the physician's income is not harmed by hospital inefficiency. That was the case under cost reimbursement. Please don't misunderstand me," he continued, "I'm not inferring that medical people are dishonest—some of the finest people I know are physicians. It's just that people respond to financial incentives—and the incentives of the traditional system were wrong."

"Interesting," Wes responded. "I've never had it explained that way before. Are there other factors that influence the cost of healthcare that I should be aware of?"

"There are," Krimmel replied. "I've set up appointments with other members of the faculty and staff that I think can best explain them to you."

10

Gaming the System?

It was 9:00 a.m. as Wes Douglas's automobile turned onto Medical Drive. This was his first visit to University Hospital. As Dr. Krimmel had a meeting scheduled, he asked Wes to drop him at the main entrance, where he gave him directions to the office of Dr. Allison Richards, Dean of the School of Medicine.

Dr. Richards, an oncologist by training, was waiting for Wes in her office. In her early fifties, Dr. Richards had silver hair, shortly tapered, and wore a white lab coat over a finely cut pant suit of gray wool. "Dr. Krimmel tells me you're here to learn about healthcare cost," she said, motioning for Wes to take a seat.

"That's true," Wes replied. He took a chair next to a large window overlooking the Moran Eye Center. "I'm especially interested in the problems caused by what Dr. Krimmel calls the *breakdown of the market mechanism* in the healthcare industry."

"It's interesting you should mention that," Richards said. Her eyes narrowed as she focused on a report she retrieved from the top drawer of his desk. "I've been studying a memo this morning from our director of reimbursement—it's a concern of his as well."

Richards thumbed to the second page. "One of the fastest-growing components of healthcare costs is diagnostic services," she said. "These include laboratory and x-ray services. While advances in technology have provided a number of valuable tools, there's growing concern a few physicians may be using them to increase personal income."

"Do you have evidence to support that conclusion?" Wes asked.

"Not at the University Hospital, although an actuary in Salt Lake City has done a study that indicates that northern Utah physicians who have ownership interests in laboratories perform significantly more tests per outpatient visit than those who don't. Her findings are consistent with studies in West Germany, where there has been a surplus of physicians. Contrary to what economists projected, increased competition has not reduced physician income—income has actually gone up."

Richards laid the report on the table and focused her eyes on Wes. "Much of the cost increase has come from an increase in outpatient x-ray and laboratory procedures."

"An eastern economist studied this phenomenon in American physicians. Concerned with the variation he found in the number of laboratory tests ordered by physicians of the same specialty in the same hospital, he was able to isolate only one variable that statistically accounted for the variance."

"What was that?" asked Wes.

"Volume—the lower the physician's patient volume, the greater his or her propensity to order unnecessary diagnostic procedures. The root of the problem is consumer ignorance. The patient doesn't know what tests he or she needs. That's why we need a methodology to provide information for regulators and consumers to use in overcoming the problem of *disparate information*. The SEC has done a good job of addressing that problem in the stock market. Unfortunately, few people have looked at it in healthcare."

"Lab and x-ray tests are not the only areas where consumer ignorance supplies an incentive for physicians to provide excessive or inappropriate services," Richards continued. "Several years ago, there was evidence we were performing too many elective surgeries. In addition, there's a strong indication that, for many years, hospitals generated excessive patient days. Ideally, hospital lenght-of-stay should be dependent solely on the patient's medical condition. Under cost reimbursement, however, there's evidence that other factors influenced the physician's discharge decision."

"Like what?" Wes asked.

"Hospital occupancy," Richards replied. "I did my residency at Community Hospital in St. Louis where we had an outstanding hospital administrator, a fellow trained at the University of Chicago. Whenever occupancy rates would dip, he would start visiting with the medical staff as they made their morning rounds. 'Doctor,' he'd say, 'remember that auto analyzer for the lab you convinced us to order last month? The one that cost $160,000? Our occupancy today is 53 percent—it sure makes it hard to justify expensive equipment with half of our beds empty.'"

Richards reflected on her experience. "Interestingly, his not-so-subtle conversations with the medical staff worked. Within a few hours the hospital census would start to climb."

"It doesn't sound like the market mechanism worked well in those days," said Wes.

"I'm not sure it worked at all," said Richards.

"What's the solution?" asked Wes.

"Some think the answer lies in incentive reimbursement," responded Richards. "That's probably the reason Dr. Krimmel scheduled Larry Ortega as your next appointment. Larry is our Director of Reimbursement."

11

Adverse Incentives

The Director of Reimbursement's office was in the basement not far from the hospital laundry. Larry Ortega was not there when Wes arrived. His secretary explained he was in negotiations with a health insurance company downtown. He had called, she said, to say he'd be a few minutes late.

Wes took a seat and, for the next fifteen minutes, thumbed through a copy of *Healthcare Financial Management.* Ortega arrived shortly after 10:00 a.m.. Earlier, the weatherman had forecast a heavy midmorning storm. From Ortega's damp appearance, Wes judged the storm had arrived.

"Sorry to be late—" Ortega said, shaking the rain from his umbrella. He unbuttoned his coat, unwrapped his muffler, and motioned for Wes to precede him into the small office that had been partitioned from a large linen room off the laundry. The hospital was obviously busy, and office space was at a premium.

At fifty-six, Ortega had a lean frame, wore a crew cut, and had a no-nonsense manner about him reminiscent of his past military training. He motioned for Wes to be seated as he checked his phone pad for messages and then looked Wes squarely in the eyes across the wooden desk that occupied most of the room.

"Herb Krimmel said you have some questions for me," he began.

Wes nodded. "Dr. Richards explained how a breakdown in what she calls the *market mechanism* can lead to the inefficient utilization of medical resources. I'm here to learn how incentive reimbursement can address that problem."

Ortega scowled as he considered the question. "If you want to learn about incentive reimbursement," he said, "you should probably know something about earlier attempts the government made to control healthcare cost." He got up from his desk and retrieved a coffeepot from a hot plate on the small credenza behind his desk.

"Coffee?" he asked.

"No thanks."

Ortega poured a cup and returned to his desk. "During the 1970s," he said, "when hospital inflation was taking off, many legislators felt the best approach to cost control was regulation. Consistent with this philosophy, they enacted laws establishing quasi-governmental agencies to review and approve requests for new hospital facilities and equipment." He paused to fan his coffee. "In some states, agencies were even established to approve hospital room rates and ancillary charges."

"That sounds like the model the government uses to regulate utilities," Wes remarked.

"I think that's what many had in mind," Ortega replied.

"It works for electric companies; how well did it work for hospitals?"

"Not well," admitted Ortega. "The problem with applying a regulation model to the healthcare industry is that, unlike utility companies which have one homogeneous product, hospitals have thousands of services and products—over 60,000 here at the University Hospital, for example. Product complexity, plus differences in the age and the severity of illness of patients treated, make it difficult for regulators to gather enough information to make intelligent decisions."

"You're telling me that central planning didn't work for healthcare for the same reason it didn't work for Eastern Europe and the former Soviet Union," Wes volunteered. "The economy's too complex for one central body to administer."

"That's right," replied Ortega. "There's little evidence that regulation did anything to control cost. If anything, it increased cost by creating a new bureaucracy within the healthcare delivery system." Ortega shook his head. "With that experience behind them, some analysts started to believe the best way to cut waste and inefficiency might be to design *incentive reimbursement systems*—systems that would encourage healthcare providers to consider cost when evaluating treatment alternatives."

"How did they plan to do that?" Wes asked, taking notes.

"By making them share in the cost of waste and inefficiency. Before 1984, most insurance plans paid hospitals their billed charges less a nominal discount. Medicare and many Medicaid plans paid cost-plus. Hospitals were reimbursed actual costs, plus a markup for profit." He smiled cynically as he placed his coffee mug on his desk. "It doesn't take a rocket scientist to find the easiest way to increase profits with a cost-plus contract."

"Increase cost!" Wes said.

"That's right. While I don't think anyone purposefully raised cost only to increase profits, strong incentives to hold the line on cost didn't exist." Ortega leaned back in his chair as he stared out the window. "When I retired from the military in 1980, I was hired as director of purchasing at Long Beach Memorial Hospital in California. I wish I had a nickel for every time an equipment vendor said: *Don't worry about the price— it's cost reimbursable under Medicare.*"

Wes's eyes reflected his bewilderment. "Cost reimbursement's not a common payment system," he reflected. "About the only other place I've seen it's in the defense industry—it's also used in some segments of the construction industry. Why was cost reimbursement the payment system of choice in healthcare?"

"The answer lies in the history of the health industry," Ortega responded. "The first insurance company in the United States was Blue Cross. This organization was formed in the 1930s by Justin Ford Kimball, a university administrator serving on the board of trustees of Baylor Hospital. As the story goes, Kimball started Blue Cross because he was concerned about the number of professors who were not paying their hospital bills. In the 1930s, most hospitals were nonprofit corporations. These were run by charitable organizations—organizations Kimball thought should be protected from financial risk. When the time came to select a payment mechanism, he chose cost reimbursement. As other insurance companies entered the healthcare market, they followed suit. That decision cost consumers billions of dollars over the next several decades."

"You're telling me that the nonprofit status of early-day hospitals influenced the selection of a payment mechanism," Wes stated.

"That's right."

"Then I guess my next question is: why were hospitals nonprofit?"

"Because they evolved from poor houses," Ortega said. "In the early part of the twentieth century, people who had family or money died at home. It was the paupers who died in charitable institutions. These poor houses were the forebearers to hospitals.

"Early hospitals were not the high-tech facilities we have today," he continued. "The first hospital in Salt Lake City was established by the Sisters of Holy Cross to care for the large number of silver miners in Park City who were dying of lead poisoning. It was an epidemic of significant proportions that lasted for many years. Do you know how they solved the problem?" he asked.

Wes shrugged. "A scientific breakthrough?" he asked.

"It was a breakthrough, all right—although I'm afraid it wasn't very scientific," Ortega answered, a smile lighting his dark blue eyes. "They got the miners to wash! Physicians finally determined that if miners would bathe more than two or three times a year, they wouldn't absorb lead from silver ore through their skin."

Ortega smiled sympathetically. "I tell that story simply to illustrate how far medicine has come. In the early part of the twentieth century, a patient had a better chance of dying if she was admitted to the hospital than if she stayed home."

Wes pondered Ortega's message. Hospitals were different in their history and incentive structure than the manufacturing firms he had been used to dealing with. He understood now why Karisa Holyoak felt he needed a better understanding of the history of the healthcare industry if he was to succeed in his new assignment.

"Okay," said Wes. "I understand why most hospitals were nonprofit organizations and how that influenced insurance companies to adopt cost reimbursement. I also understand how cost reimbursement destroyed incentives for cost control available to other industries. My next question is—what's the alternative?"

"Some think it's incentive reimbursement," replied Ortega.

"Is that the same as prospective payment?" Wes asked.

"A prospective payment system is one form of incentive reimbursement, as you may know. A prospective payment system is one where an insurance company negotiates a fixed price for a predefined set of medical goods and services prior to the onset of a patient's illness. In the terminology of contracting—it's a fixed-price contract."

Wes nodded. "I understand the terminology. When I was in college, I worked part time as an accountant for a building contractor. Some of his projects were built under fixed-price contracts; others he built on a cost-reimbursement basis."

"Do you think he managed them the same?" asked Ortega.

"I'd like to say he did, but I have to admit there was more pressure to control cost on fixed-price contracts than there was under the cost-reimbursement contracts."

"Why was that?" Ortega asked.

"Fixed-price contracts place the contractor at risk; cost-reimbursement contracts don't."

"That's right," replied Ortega. "Most people are less careful when spending other people's money than they are when spending their own. The same principle holds true for healthcare," he continued. "Physicians had little to lose if hospital resources were used inefficiently, and since hospitals were reimbursed for inefficient care, hospitals didn't have much to lose either."

Ortega leaned back in his chair as he studied Wes Douglas. *Wes is a bright enough fellow, but he still has a lot to learn*, he thought. "I think the best person to explain how prospective payment systems can change physician behavior is Charles Stoker, the

Director of our new HMO. He's out of town today, but he'll be back later this week. I could set up an appointment if you'd like."

"That would be great," answered Wes. "It will give me a chance to get back to the hospital this afternoon and take care of the items on my desk."

12

Amy

It was noon when Wes returned to the hospital. Birdie Bankhead was leaving for lunch when he met her in the employee parking lot. "There are several messages on your desk," she said, fishing in her purse for her keys. "The bank called. You left the hospital's copy of the note in Whittingham's office—they will mail it to you."

"The bank has renewed the note on the condition the hospital be at break-even within ninety days," Wes replied. "I must get with the department heads to formulate a plan."

Birdie looked at him sympathetically. "Won't be easy," she said. "Budgeting never was one of Hap's strengths. I anticipate you'll meet with some resistance from the staff."

Wes shrugged.

Birdie's eyes widened with recollection. "That reminds me," she said. "Hap's daughter Amy came by this morning to clean out his office. She's still there. You'll enjoy meeting her."

Wes nodded and headed for the employee entrance. By now everyone recognized him as the new administrator. Just navigating from the parking lot to Administration was a difficult chore, as physicians, supervisors, and employees collared him to voice complaints and give advice. It took twenty minutes from the time he entered the building before he arrived safely at Administration.

By the time he reached his office, his arms were full of three-ring binders containing past minutes of the Tissue, Infections, and Credentials Committees that the secretary of the medical staff had asked him to review and sign. Nudging the door leading from the hall to Birdie's office closed, he leaned against it momentarily as he caught his breath and then deposited the binders on Birdie's desk.

With all the interruptions, he had forgotten about Amy Castleton. He was surprised when, through the door of Hap's old office, he saw her reading from a stack of papers on the massive walnut desk. Her head was turned gently to one side, exposing a slender white neck. She had long, amber hair that glowed softly in the sunlight that poured through the French doors leading to the patio. Mute, he stared at her as she read from a letter she had picked up from Hap's desk. She looked up, startled.

"Hi," he said, "I'm Wes Douglas. "

Pursing her lips, she studied him for a moment—then her eyes lit with recognition. "Wes Douglas—of course . . . Father's new financial consultant," she hesitated, "and now his replacement." She smiled sadly and held out her hand. Wes gently shook it as he sat in the chair next to hers.

"Dad was pleased with your decision to consult with the hospital," she said. "I'm sorry you didn't have more time to work together."

"I'm sorry too, we will miss your father," he said gently.

A shadow crossed Amy's face and her brown eyes filled with tears. Looking down at the letter she was holding, she bit softly on her lower lip. Wes Douglas hadn't felt clumsy around a girl since he had fallen in love with Carol Reimschussel in the eighth grade. To his surprise, that awkward feeling had suddenly returned.

As he stared into her eyes, an unfamiliar intensity overcame him. It took a moment for him to realize he was still holding—squeezing actually—her hand. She looked at their hands and then into his face. A questioning look stole across her eyes. Blushing, he released her hand. Anxious to start anew, he pointed to a picture on the desk, which Amy had removed from the wall above the credenza. "That's an interesting painting," he said. "I noticed it when I first met your father—is it yours?"

Color touched her cheeks. She smiled and nodded. "I painted it when I was four years old," she stated lifting it off the desk. "Dad framed and hung it in his office—at that age I was so proud."

Her eyes, soft and sentimental, slowly surveyed the room. "Some of my happiest hours were spent here with Dad on Saturday mornings," she said. "Mom was taking a class at the university, and he would bring me with him while he opened the mail and caught up on correspondence. Sometimes I'd paint."

The picture, painted with colorful acrylics, measured six by eight inches and was framed in walnut to match the paneling of the office. A drawing of a large man holding three balloons dominated the picture. At his side was a small girl holding a flower. A huge tree, the sun, flowers, chipmunks, and stop signs, in all their profusion of color, filled the remaining white space.

"Those were all the things I knew how to draw at that age," she explained, an impish smile playing at the corners of her mouth.

"Dad wasn't given much to worrying," she said, "but during the last few weeks of his life, he changed." Her eyes narrowed as she searched for the right words. "He acted as though something were wrong, but he wouldn't talk about it. He was never one to give much attention to his health," she continued, "but six weeks before the accident he took out a life-insurance policy—I wonder if he knew something was going to happen to him."

"People sometimes have premonitions," Wes said.

"We had hoped the fishing trip would restore his old enthusiasm," Amy said sadly. "He seemed so tired—" Neither spoke as she examined the belongings she had removed from his desk.

"I was finishing when you came in," she said presently. "In a few more minutes I'll have all of Dad's things, but I can come back later if you need to use the office."

"There's no rush," he said. "I was headed out. Take your time."

Amy's eyes softened as she shook her head and smiled. "I hope you will visit us," she said. "I know Mother would enjoy meeting you."

He nodded and turned to leave. As he did, her hand gently brushed his, and as he walked to the parking lot, he wondered if it was intentional and if there was something else she had wanted to tell him.

* * *

By now Wes Douglas was settling into a routine. Often, in the evenings he would get up on the floors. It was a good chance to meet employees and talk to patients. Both were a good source of suggestions. One patient had asked for a clock in the room so she would know when to take her medications. Wes decided that if he ever built a hospital, each room would have a clock. The food carts were noisy, especially early in the morning when some patients were still trying to sleep. He would visit with the Dietary Department to see if the transportation aides could be more careful.

"Could you invent a hospital gown that was modest?" a young executive queried. It was a good idea, from his own experience as a patient Wes remembered having to hold the back of his gown together when he walked down the hall to keep from exposing his backside.

"I was cold when they wheeled me to radiology for tests," a patient reported. Henceforth, patients transported on carts through the hospital would not only be gowned but would have the warmth and privacy of cotton blanket.

"Ever taken ride through the hospital on your back on a gurney?" a patient asked. Wes's curiosity was piqued. He tried it. The next morning Housekeeping had orders to wash the ceilings and remove cobwebs from light fixtures and hallway corners vertical people didn't see.

A sociologist from the University of Wyoming was admitted after a hiking accident. Wes spent an hour visiting with him one evening, listening to his observations.

"Your hospital has a way of dehumanizing people," the professor said, "of stripping them of their personal identity. You replace their clothes with a generic gown. Their jewelry, and anything else that differentiates them from others, is impounded. Your nurses ignore patients names, referring to them as *the gallbladder in room 247* or the *hip replacement in room 312.* Your Admissions Department goes one step further, replacing their name with a number stamped on a banal plastic bracelet and tied around their wrist as though they were an infant. The staff won't trust a patient to tell them who they are, they have to check the bracelet."

Wes wrote each of the sociologist's observations down. If they survived the financial crisis, he would find ways to humanize the hospital experience.

* * *

The next evening Wes decided that he would visit patients on the second floor. As he exited the elevator, the first person he saw was a ten-year old boy in a wheelchair. Not seriously injured, he obviously had done something bizarre—the expression on his face was comical and his appearance was extraordinary. Both his legs were in casts, both hands were bandaged, his hair was singed and his eyelashes were gone.

Wes smiled as he remembered how easy it had been to get into trouble at age ten. One of these days he'd have to apologize for all of the anxiety he and his younger brother had put their parents through.

"What did *you* do?" he asked curiously.

"I climbed a power pole to catch a bird," he replied with a dazed expression. He was quiet for a moment as he remembered the experience. "When I touched the pole," he said slowly, "I stayed in the air . . . but my body dropped. I watched it fall . . ." His singed eyebrows rose in astonishment. "When it hit the fence," he said, "I went back into it."

The young man looked up at Wes as though he expected him to answer a question he himself wasn't old enough to put into words. Wes was silent as he studied the boy quietly, not exactly sure how to respond. Finally he nodded. "Well," he said, his voice soft but upbeat, "We're glad you're back!"

In the first room off the elevator was a sixteen-year old boy with spiked green hair, a tattoo, and three body piercings. Since his admission, the patient oscillated between ominous silence and violent rage. A drug user, he had been admitted the previous evening with his second case of hepatitis thanks to dirty needles.

"Keep this up," his physician said, "and you'll die."

"I don't give a _____," the youth replied.

Wes had visited only once. The young man ejected him with a volley of profanity. Wes understood that his physician was ordering a psychiatric consult. Wes continued down the hall, hopeful that the staff could help the boy resolve his problems before it was too late.

In the next room, in a circle electric bed, was a young police officer from Heber. The patient's name was Don Hemphill. There had been a problem with his insurance that the hospital's business office had originally mishandled. Alerted by the nursing staff, Wes visited him a week earlier to apologize. Wes had returned on four other occasions and they had become friends.

Hemphill was thirty-two years old, the same age as Wes but had a wife and two little blonde girls, one four and one six, who visited him every evening. They were there this evening, in bright red dresses that matched valentines they were giving their father—never mind that it was October.

Wes had discussed the case with Dr. Allen McBride, the hospital's neurologist. The patient had an ependymoma—cancer of the spinal cord. Dr. McBride explained that that the cancer had arisen in the enendymal cells of the central canal. As the ventral side of the spinal cord contains the alpha motor neurons that control voluntary muscle movement, the young man was now paralyzed.

Earlier that afternoon Wes had gone to Don's room to announce that the insurance problem had been resolved. Don showed Wes the latest picture of his daughters. "God has been good to me," he said smiling. "I'm going to beat this you know." Wes admired his optimism, but Don was wrong. An hour later the doctors informed Connie Hemphill that Don's condition was terminal; he would be dead by February. That afternoon, Connie retrieved love notes her daughters had made but were saving for their daddy—hence, the valentines in October.

Wes paused in the doorway outside, not wanting to interrupt. His expression grew stilled and serious. *I don't' understand. In room 201 we have a teenager who has given himself hepatitis—twice. He is trying to throw his life away, says he doesn't care if he survives—but he will. In the next room is a young father who wants so desperately to live—but he won't.*

As he continued down the hall, he realized that hospital administrators were confronted on a daily basis with issues for which a business degree provided little, if any, preparation.

13

Is There a Solution?

Charles Stoker stood five foot eight and had a full head of wavy white hair that bestowed a patrician-like appearance. A former hospital administrator, Stoker had been hired to organize the hospital's first health maintenance organization, more commonly called an HMO. It was Wes Douglas's second day at University Hospital, and he was back to learn more about hospital cost control.

"I've seen three major revolutions in the healthcare industry in my lifetime," said Stoker. "The first one occurred in the 1970s with the consolidation of hospitals into corporate chains. It was a difficult time for many hospital administrators who had grown accustomed to the autonomy and, in some cases, the lack of accountability of the old system." Wes took notes.

"The second revolution," Stoker continued, "took place in the 1980s with the introduction of prospective payment systems. Cost reimbursement placed little risk on healthcare providers and encouraged over utilization and waste in some cases. It was difficult for administrators who had grown up in a no risk environment to change the way they did business. Many basic assumptions of hospital operations changed."

"The third revolution occurred in the 1990s as more and more providers assumed an insurance role, bypassing insurance companies and contracting directly with employers for the provision of comprehensive health services."

Wes shot Stoker a questioning look. "Why would a provider willingly assume the economic risk that the formation of an insurance entity entails?"

"Two reasons," Stoker replied. "Market share's the first. Prospective payment has placed a limit on the growth of hospital revenue. It caps payments and limits lenght-of-stay. The only way for hospitals to increase revenue is to capture additional patients," he explained.

"Captive health plans allow hospitals to do that by dictating to employees what physicians they must use to get maximum discounts," Stoker continued, "and by controlling the hospital admission patterns of participating physicians."

"And the second?" Wes queried.

"Cost control. One of the most effective provider insurance organizations is the health maintenance organization, often called the HMO." Stoker retrieved a plan description and handed it to Wes.

"That's what I was hired to organize here at the University Hospital," Stoker said. "This document describes our plan."

"Are health-maintenance organizations a recent development?" Wes asked paging through the brochure.

"Yes and no," Stoker replied. "The first HMO in the country was formed in the 1940s by an industrialist named Henry Kaiser. Kaiser had a contract to build ships for the war effort. In an effort to recruit employees without violating wage controls, he began offering his employees health benefits. His program used a prospective payment system called *capitation payment.*"

"What's that?" Wes asked.

"A capitation payment system is one in which the healthcare provider receives a fixed amount per patient per month to provide a set of specified services, often full comprehensive inpatient and outpatient healthcare services. The doctor and the hospital receive this amount, regardless of whether the patient uses services or not."

"How does that help?" asked Wes.

"It provides an incentive to keep the patient well," Stoker said. "And if the patient becomes ill, it encourages the physician to use the most cost-effective resources to get him or her better. The incentive to cure the patient's still there—the threat of malpractice and the ability of employers to shop for health insurance companies provides that mechanism. Also, poorly treated patients get sicker and use more healthcare resources. Unlike fee-for-service or cost-reimbursement payment systems, however, capitation payment does not provide an incentive for the physician to over-utilize products and services."

Stoker studied Wes. It was obvious he didn't understand. "Let me give you an example I often share with employers when I'm marketing our plan," Stoker continued. "Role play with me. Assume you are an obstetrician at Peter Brannan Community Hospital. Last Friday, one of your patients came in, and you delivered a baby. It's Monday morning, and you're up on the floor doing rounds. As you are writing her discharge orders, she says something like this:

I have a small problem, Dr. Douglas. My husband can't get off work to help me with the baby and so my mother's flying in from Seattle to give me a hand. Unfortunately, she can't get off work 'till Wednesday. How about letting me stay in the hospital until then? My husband works at the steel plant where he's insured by Blue Cross's traditional indemnity plan—it will pay all of the additional cost.

Wes wrinkled his brow. "What's an indemnity plan?" he asked.

"An indemnity insurance plan is one that places no limit on the care that can be provided, usually does no peer or utilization review, and pays the hospital charges or discounted charges," Stoker replied. "You are the doctor, Wes. If you say no to her request, what do you have to lose?"

"Her goodwill," said Wes. "She might change doctors. Worse still, she might bad-mouth me to her neighbors or friends, which would cause me to lose additional patients."

"That's right," Stoker said smiling. "Now let's look and see what you win if you say *yes.*"

"I retain her goodwill," Wes said. "By keeping her in a few more days, I might even make more money."

Stoker nodded approvingly. "Now let's talk about the other stakeholders in your decision. Let's start with the hospital. Remember now—this is a traditional insurance program—hospitals are still under cost reimbursement."

Wes rubbed his chin as he stared at the ceiling. "Well—the hospital administrator will probably be happy," he said. "A longer lenght-of-stay increases cost and hospital reimbursement."

"That's right," said Stoker, his eyes flashing approval. "How about the insurance company?"

"I'm not sure . . ." said Wes.

"In the 1970s, they didn't care," said Stoker. "Most health insurers felt their role was that of intermediary, or bill payer. Insurance companies simply passed the additional cost to the employer in increased premiums. Rarely did they question utilization or provider charges."

"What about the employer?" asked Wes. "He couldn't be too happy about my decision to leave her in three more days. Eventually, he would have to pay the bill through higher premiums"

"That's true," said Stoker, "but he was so far removed from the decision he had little to say in the matter."

"You're telling me the same thing Krimmel said—cost reimbursement provided few incentives for cost control."

"That's what I'm saying," said Stoker. "Now let's talk about economic incentives under a capitation payment system. Let's assume now that you're a physician who has been hired by an organization that receives a capitation payment—an HMO." Stoker paused to collect his thoughts as he developed this scenario.

"Let's say I'm the medical director of the organization," he continued, "and this is your first day on the job. The morning you start seeing patients I call you into my office and say something like this:

Dr. Douglas, we're glad to have you on board. Your references are excellent, and I think you'll find this is a good place to work. Before you begin seeing patients, however, let me tell you how we're going to pay you. Your compensation has two components. You will receive a base salary and a bonus. Your bonus will be paid at the end of the year and may run anywhere from zero to 200 percent of your salary, depending on how much money our HMO has left at the end of the year from the premiums we collect from employers.

We receive $125 per month for every enrollee in our HMO. For this $125 we provide all the health services the patient requires, including office visits, laboratory and x-ray tests, prescriptions, physical therapy, and hospitalization. If the patient uses no services during the month, we get $125 from his or her employer. If the patient uses $100,000 of healthcare services, we still get $125.

Bonuses come from the premium pool left after expenses are paid. Our physicians get 80 percent of those profits; the remainder is retained by the HMO to buy equipment, provide working capital, and pay for possible losses.

"I think I understand the system," said Wes. "If resources are used inefficiently, it's the HMO that loses—not the patient or employer. That changes the incentive of the physician, doesn't it?"

"You bet it does," said Stoker. "Let me put you in my time machine and take you back to that fictitious maternity patient. This time let's assume she's insured by our HMO." Stoker smiled menacingly. "Now tell me what each of the stakeholders has to win or lose."

Wes's eyes narrowed as he mulled the question. "Well," he said, "as an HMO physician, I would be reluctant to leave her in the hospital if the additional days were not medically justified."

"Why?" Stoker asked.

"Because two additional days would reduce year-end profits, and my year-end bonus."

"That's right," said Stoker. "What about the hospital administrator—how would she feel about the decision to leave the patient in the hospital longer than medically necessary?"

"If her institution's being paid under capitation payment, she no longer has an incentive to increase patient days—keeping the patient longer would reduce hospital profits."

"And the insurance company?"

"If employers are managing their employee healthcare cost more aggressively, as you have indicated, then they probably would shop on the basis of price as well as quality—the HMO would have an incentive to monitor hospital costs, which would reflect in premiums."

"What about the employer?" Stoker asked.

"He would be happy. For the first time there would be an incentive for the healthcare provider to make cost-effective decisions."

Wes's eyes flashed with skepticism. "Sounds good in theory—but are HMOs more cost effective than traditional insurance programs?"

"There's evidence they are," said Stoker. "One of the major components of healthcare cost is hospitalization. Local studies indicate that participants in indemnity plans generate 300 to 400 patient days per year per 1,000 enrollees. HMOs generate 220. Some companies I talk to estimate they have reduced their employee healthcare cost by as much as 25 percent since enrolling their employees in HMOs."

"That's good for the employer," Wes said, "but what does it do to a hospital like mine that depends on a longer lenght-of-stay to maintain patient volumes?"

"It provides a strong incentive to control cost," Stoker replied.

"If HMOs work so well, why didn't they take off back in the 1940s when Henry Kaiser started the prototype? Prior to 1985, I'd never heard of an HMO," Wes said.

"For many years, medical associations were effective in shutting them down," said Stoker. "When I was a healthcare administration student in Seattle, there was a physician in the inner city who started charging his patients on a capitation basis. The Washington Medical Association tried to get him thrown in prison for violating state insurance laws—laws they had helped draft, laws designed to keep HMOs out of the state."

"One of the most aggressive medical associations in the country was the Oregon Medical Association," Stoker continued. "It persuaded the legislature to pass a law that HMOs could keep none of their surpluses but had to absorb all losses. It was a law designed to force HMOs into insolvency—which it did.

"In other areas of the country, state medical associations prohibited physicians who worked for HMOs from joining their organizations. Hospital bylaws were then modified to prohibit doctors who were not members of local medical associations from joining hospital medical staffs. As a result, HMO physicians were excluded from hospital practice."

"What happened to change that trend?" Wes asked.

"In the early 1980s, the Federal Government passed legislation overriding all of the anti-HMO laws state legislatures had enacted through the years. The effect of that legislation on the growth of capitated insurance plans was astounding" Stoker said.

"Are there other prospective payment systems?" Wes asked.

"DRG reimbursement," Stoker replied—"It stands *for Diagnostic Group Reimbursement.*"

"A mouthful," said Wes.

"Sure is," replied Stoker. "DRG is a form of prospective payment. Under capitation payment, the hospital receives a fixed payment per enrollee per month, regardless of the services rendered. Under DRG reimbursement, it receives a fixed payment per *Diagnosis-Related Group.*"

"I'm not sure I understand," said Wes, "what's a diagnosis-related group?"

"A diagnosis-related group is a disease classification. When a patient's discharged from Peter Brannan Community Hospital, he or she is assigned a DRG based on the discharge diagnosis. Say for example, that a sixty-five-year-old female is discharged with a diagnosis of rheumatic pericarditis. Her case would be assigned to DRG 393. The hospital would receive $8,670 for her treatment. That $8,670 would be fixed. It wouldn't matter how long she stayed in the hospital or what products and services she received; the hospital would only get $8,670."

"I imagine DRG reimbursement had a dramatic effect on average lenght-of-stay," observed Wes.

"It did," replied Stoker. "Prior to the introduction of DRG reimbursement, the national average lenght-of-stay was about thirteen days. In Utah, it was about seven— we have a younger population and didn't have as many excess hospital beds to fill. When DRG reimbursement took effect, the national average dropped to seven days. Utah's dropped to 3.5."

"How do efficient hospitals prosper under DRG reimbursement?" Wes asked.

"They control cost." Stoker said. "That's why there is so much current emphasis on cost accounting for the purpose of cost control."

"What keeps the hospital from providing less care than needed to get the patient well?" Wes asked.

"I'm not sure I have a complete answer to that," Stoker replied. "The threat of a malpractice suit plays a role. If the patient gets sicker while in the hospital, and has to stay longer, the hospital loses money. Also, if discharged patients are readmitted within a short period, the hospital receives no reimbursement for the second admission."

"It sounds like the new environment requires a new management style," Wes said.

"That's true," said Stoker. "Shortly after managed care was introduced, 30 percent of the hospital administrators in the country lost their jobs. Many couldn't adjust to an entirely new set of assumptions, one of the most dramatic being that under capitation payment, an empty bed is a profitable bed. If Peter Brannan Community

Hospital is to survive," he continued, "it will have to change the way it does business. Making the necessary changes won't be easy. Physicians and managers who are comfortable with the old system will resist them. Your task will be to make those changes—without getting canned."

Wes nodded warily.

* * *

Driving back to apartment that evening, Wes reflected on what he had learned about healthcare cost and the steps being taken by government and industry to stem the tide of inflation. His conversation with Stoker on prospective payment system clarified the issues discussed in his first meeting with the board.

It was apparent that Hap and his administrative team had not anticipated the dramatic way prospective payment would influence the operation of the hospital. Under a cost-reimbursement system, the hospital made money by admitting many patients, keeping them a long time, and providing as many ancillary services as possible.

DRG reimbursement changed the equation. Hospitals still made money by admitting patients. Since reimbursement per admission was fixed, however, the financial incentive was to provide only those services necessary to cure patients, discharging them as quickly as possible.

Capitation payment changed the equation even further. Here hospitals made money by keeping patients out of the hospital altogether—the emphasis was clearly on prevention. Prior to prospective payment, hospitals had never been in the healthcare business—they were in the *sick-care* business.

Under cost reimbursement, hospitals and physicians made money only when patients got sick. Now, under capitation payment, it was to the economic benefit of the participating hospital and physician to prevent illness before it consumed provider resources.

If successful, capitation payment had the potential to create a *healthcare* rather than a *sick-care* system. Wes liked the emphasis. *How does a hospital make money at it though? Good contracts with HMOs, low utilization—an emphasis on prevention,* he thought, answering his own question. *We must change our strategy!*

Wes now understood why physicians like Dr. Flagg felt threatened by the changes taking place in the healthcare industry. Under cost reimbursement, the physicians who admitted many patients, kept them in the hospital for long periods of time, and used high quantities of ancillary services were heroes to the hospital administrator.

With the adoption of prospective payment, high-resource consumers suddenly became villains. Retraining physicians in the new model would not be easy, especially during the present transition period from fee-for-service and cost reimbursement to prospective payment systems.

Although the economics of incentive reimbursement made sense, there was another issue that bothered Wes—quality. *"Under capitation payment, what's to prevent physicians from providing too little care or too few services?"* Flagg had asked. *"We've got obstetric patients being discharged the same day as the delivery—I'm uncomfortable with that practice,"* he had continued.

There were other quality issues as well. Dr. Flagg was concerned that the current environment was causing hospitals to cut staffing to levels that jeopardized the safety of hospital care. Wes could understand how that could happen. Although the threat of malpractice theoretically mitigated economic misbehavior, the possibility still troubled Flagg. It troubled Wes, too.

Maybe Flagg's behavior is understandable. He was raised in an era that rewarded independent thought and action. That wasn't all bad. HMOs with their pre-certification, utilization review panels, and salaried physicians are changing all that.

Wes heard rumors of hospital systems that were bullying physicians into selling their practices. *"Sell your practice and join us as an employee, or we'll build a clinic across the street and put you out of business."* In the old days, private-practice physicians were the hospital's valued customers. In a staff model HMO environment they became the competition.

Wes shook his head as he thought about the conflicting forces he would have to contend with as the new administrator of Peter Brannan Community Hospital—physicians who wanted more equipment, a board that wanted lower cost, and patients who expected the hospital to save them *"at any cost,"* but not bill them. Hospital administration was not an easy job.

14

The Robbery

"Whoever broke in must have known what they were after," said Sergeant Peter O'Malley, rubbing the scruff of his morning beard with the back of his large, beefy hand. O'Malley hadn't shaved yet—the call from hospital security came just as he was getting into the shower.

O'Malley was an old-time cop—one who made an effort to know everyone on his beat. Park City was not only safer, but was a friendlier place because of O'Malley. The sergeant was physically well endowed for the part. With his red curly hair and large beer belly, he looked like a character from a Norman Rockwell painting.

O'Malley's eyes, a curious shade of green, swept the room for additional clues. "Whatever they wanted, it wasn't money. The cash drawer's intact—the safe wasn't even touched." He shook his head as he studied an old desk in the corner next to a large window. "What they wanted was here," he said with a generous sweep of his arm.

Moving to the desk, he removed a small magnifying glass from his shirt pocket and examined the broken lock on the file drawer. The surface had been dusted for fingerprints—none had been found. Finished, he tucked the magnifier back into his pocket. "Prints were wiped clean," he sniffed. "Who does it belong to?"

Kayla Elmore, the accounts receivables clerk, stepped forward. "It's Del Cluff's desk," she said, her eyes wide with wonder. Robberies were not common in Park City.

"Did he keep any valuables in it?" O'Malley asked.

"I doubt it," she said softly, "he didn't have any valuables." Several employees laughed. Mr. Cluff came to work looking like a Bavarian peasant—his ill-fitting suits were Goodwill Industry specials. He lived in a rented room two blocks from Main Street and drove a battered Volkswagen bus.

"No—Del Cluff probably didn't have any valuables," an accountant volunteered.

Kayla's smoky blue eyes sobered as she studied the battered desk. "It hasn't been opened since the accident," she continued looking up at O'Malley. "Mr. Cluff's still in a coma at University Hospital—we don't have a second key."

O'Malley examined the desk. It was open *now*. A crowbar had been used to pry the lock off the file drawer. Its contents had been dumped on the gray linoleum floor. O'Malley was silent as he finished an incident report attached to his clipboard.

"With no suspects, and no idea of what—if anything—was taken, there's not much more I can do," he said. He signed the report with a flourish and handed it to Natalie Simpson, who had been appointed acting controller. "Initial here, and I'll file a report with the department."

Natalie initialed the form and handed it back to O'Malley. Natalie turned to examine the desk once more, shot a glance at Wes Douglas, who had come for his nine o'clock appointment, and shrugged.

"This is the first time in my recollection we've had a burglary—and to think all they got was a bunch of old files," O'Malley said. His face exploded in a grin. "At least they didn't get the payroll—that's all this new Douglas fellow would have needed." Several employees laughed. By now the entire community was aware of the hospital's precarious situation.

Satisfied the investigation was over, Natalie Simpson retrieved an armful of folders from the floor and dumped them on Del Cluff's desk. Others followed suit. While the other employees continued to clean up, Natalie grabbed Wes by the arm and led him into the hall. They had an appointment to review the hospital's latest financial reports. "If you still want to meet," she said, "we can use the conference room."

"Got a better idea," said Wes. "I need your signature on a note at the bank. Let's take care of that. While we're out, you can show me the property Wycoff wants the lien on. Any additional agenda items can be covered as we drive."

*　*　*

The paperwork took less than five minutes to complete. The bank president was so happy to have Wycoff assume financial responsibility for the hospital's $2 million line of credit that he almost offered Wes free checking on his personal account. Instead, he gave him a plastic ballpoint pen with the bank's name and his picture printed prominently on the side.

Five minutes later, Wes's Taurus was turning north on the old highway leaving Park City. "What happened to Selman?" Wes asked as his car merged with traffic.

"Caught in the middle," Natalie replied. "Hap didn't like him because he was too financially conservative. Edward Wycoff didn't trust him because he wasn't conservative enough. The issue came to a head during the negotiations for the new hospital.

"Hap realized the competition would eventually capture our market if we didn't replace the outdated facility. He was too ambitious, however. He wanted to build too many beds—to grow the business too fast. Wycoff recognized that prospective payment would limit the hospital's ability to recover new capital expenditures. He was unwilling to approve a significant outlay without a clear understanding of how it would be recovered. Both viewpoints, taken to the extreme, would have spelled disaster for the hospital. Selman tried to play the middle ground and, as a result, wound up alienating both sides."

"Old Chinese saying—*Man who walks in middle of road gets hit by cars going both ways,*" Wes said.

Natalie smiled and nodded. "Appropriate observation. Hap didn't value Selman's judgment. He was an optimist and didn't like the things his controller had to tell him. Despite that, Selman remained loyal to Hap, even when it hurt his relationship with Wycoff."

"Why?" Wes asked.

"Three years ago, Selman's wife was diagnosed with breast cancer. Selman was pretty upset about it and wasn't paying attention to business. It was the end of the fiscal year, and the hospital was changing its funding mechanism for the employee health insurance plan, converting from a fully insured to self insured plan. Over ten years it had accumulated $600,000 of savings, held in a special fund by the company."

"Since it was a mutual insurance company, the hospital was technically entitled to 80% of that fund. In the new contract, the insurance company nullified the hospital's right to that money. Selman signed without picking up on that clause. It cost the hospital almost a half million dollars."

Wes whistled. "Painful mistake."

Natalie nodded. "Wycoff found out about it and went through the ceiling. He went to the board and demanded Selman's dismissal. Hap, aware of the turmoil Selman was experiencing, stepped in, taking blame for the mistake himself.

"Hap was more popular with the board and medical staff then," Natalie continued. "Wycoff didn't have the strength to oust him, so Selman kept his job. Selman never forgot it."

Wes's eyes darkened. "That explains why Wycoff moved so quickly in firing Selman after Hap died," he said. "He was just settling an old score."

Natalie gave Wes a side look. "You're probably right. You have to understand that Wycoff did many of the right things, though often for the wrong reasons. He was brilliant, but ruthless—people didn't mean anything to him."

"Hap, on the other hand, did a lot of things that didn't make sense from a business standpoint. However, there was never a doubt of his loyalty to the patients, or his employees. He was stubborn, sometimes even prideful—but he cared about people, and the employees loved him for it. Even with managed care, he believed that hospitals should still act like charitable institutions.

Wes understood. "When the public started demanding a *bottom-line approach* to hospital management," he said, "the industry lost some of the characteristics that made it special."

Natalie sighed. "It's a different game today. In the old days, the purpose was to heal the patient, regardless of the cost or the patient's ability to pay. Hospitals were often inefficient and sometimes outright wasteful, but they cooperated with each other in achieving that objective. Today, the objective for many administrators is to reduce cost and save money, even when physicians, employees, and patients are treated less than honorably."

"Let's hope they'll reach a balance between efficiency and empathy," Wes said.

"Some are there already. For others, it will take longer."

Less than a mile north of Highway 40, Natalie motioned for her boss to stop the car. Wes pulled off the road. About six hundred yards up a gradual hill, a chain-link fence enclosed the abandoned site. The construction equipment was gone, all that remained were the footings, a pile of bricks, and two stacks of rebar.

"That's the project?" Wes asked in surprise.

Natalie nodded. They left the car, climbing the hill in long lumbering steps.

"Our property runs from the fence to the top of the hill," Natalie pointed east. "One hundred acres in all, purchased in 1993. There were to be three construction phases. Phase one was the physicians' office building; phase two the outpatient facility; phase three patient rooms and supporting departments.

"The project was to be financed by industrial revenue bonds underwritten by Park City State Bank. Back then the bank was owned by the Brannan family. The Mike and Sara Brannan Foundation pledged an additional million dollars."

"Neat package, too bad it didn't work," Wes said.

"When the Brannan empire unraveled, so did the new hospital," Natalie replied.

Wes was impressed with the area. The property was easily accessible from the freeway. Power and water were already on the site. "How much of the land was needed for the hospital?" he asked.

"The three phases, would have occupied thirty-five acres," Natalie responded. "The rest was for future development. Rumor has it a group from back east would like to buy the property for a hotel complex. If we sold it, we could get triple what we paid for it. A better option would be to build a new hospital on it."

A black Lincoln Continental crested the hill and stopped. Two men exited. One of them pointed to a barbed-wire fence that bordered the property on the north. "Looks like Wycoff's car," Natalie said.

Wes opened his car door and retrieved a set of binoculars from under the seat. "It is," he said focusing. "Who's that with him?"

Wes passed the glasses to Natalie. Natalie was silent as she adjusted the focus. "Tony Devecchi." she said. "Wycoff brought him to Kiwanis last week. He's a retired businessman from Arizona. Owns a chain of nursing homes. He's been kicking around town for a couple of weeks. Probably looking for a place to retire."

"What's he doing with Wycoff?" Wes asked.

"Want to ask him?"

"Nope, it's time to get home. If he's got money, Wycoff's probably setting him up for a contribution."

✻ ✻ ✻

Wes was quiet on the drive back to the hospital. The discussion about Edward Wycoff and his relationship with Roger Selman had re-alerted him to the power struggle within the board. Wes was aware of the conflict when he accepted the job. Back then, however, he believed that most of the issues were black and white. Now he was starting to see a lot of gray.

Castleton, Wycoff, Brannan, and the medical staff had been at war. Castleton was gone, but the others remained. In the beginning, Wes thought the battle was over efficiency—the good guys were for lower cost and higher quality care; the bad guys were for the inefficient status quo. Wes now saw that the stakes involved more than money and power. Issues of quality, compassion, and even integrity were starting to muddy the waters.

Maybe the opponents in this battle didn't wear black and white hats—perhaps they all wore gray. Wes wasn't sure. What he did know was that it was becoming increasingly difficult for him to identify exclusively with either of the two viewpoints.

Wycoff knew what was best financially, but had forgotten that healthcare was about people. Hap's heart was in the right place, but his hostility to accountants and efficiency experts hampered his ability to control costs.

What value is high-quality care if no one can afford it? Wes didn't blame Hap for not cutting costs in areas that would reduce accessibility or quality. He did blame him, however, for refusing to adopt efficiencies that could have avoided the crisis Peter Brannan Community Hospital faced.

Wes frowned. *And then there's Wycoff—what's he up to? Is he trying to help a hospital that was nurtured for a generation by the philanthropy of the Brannan family, or does he have other motives?* Wes believed the former, but skepticism on the part of the medical staff made him uncertain.

✱ ✱ ✱

When Wes returned to the hospital that afternoon, there was a note on his desk that Kayla Elmore, the Accounts Receivables Clerk, wanted to see him. He called for her to come down.

Kayla was smiling with satisfaction as she entered his office. "I think I know what the robber took," she said handing him a folder. "This was on the floor along with all the other stuff from Del's desk. It's empty now; it wasn't when Cluff had me type the label."

Wes took the folder, the label read: *Internal Audit—Pharmacy.*

"Did you read what was inside?"

"Nope, just typed the label. When I saw it on the floor, empty and all, I thought it might be important."

"Might be," Wes affirmed. "Thanks for your diligence, Kayla."

Kayla grinned at the praise.

15

The Hospital Bazaar

It was ten o'clock Saturday. *Time for a break*, Wes thought as he stretched the knots out of his back. Inhaling deeply, he pushed the chair away from his desk, piled high with paper. Crossing his office, he locked the doors and was exiting to the lobby when he heard a familiar voice. Turning, he saw Amy Castleton.

"A little higher, Niels, and to the right," she said, motioning gently with both hands. Three feet above on a metal ladder, sixty-one-year-old Niels Svendsen, senior custodian, obediently re-hung a poster on the freshly painted wall.

Wrinkling her brow, she studied the new location and then smiled with satisfaction. "That'll do it!" She smiled brightly.

"Finally," Niels gasped good-naturedly. Removing a roll of tape from his worn coveralls, he attached the poster securely. It advertised the auxiliary bazaar to be held that afternoon at Canyon Park.

Petite and flower-like, Amy wore a pink cotton volunteer's uniform that defined the narrowness of her waist. As Niels teased her, she laughed, tossing her head to the side so that her thick, auburn hair bounced on her shoulders. Turning to take another poster down the hall, she ran headlong into Wes. "Excuse me!" she gasped. "Didn't know you were there."

She stepped back embarrassed; he struggled not to blush. It was not every day he had a beautiful girl run into his arms. Tongue tied, he pointed at the poster. "Must be the hospital bazaar today?" He was immediately embarrassed by the dumbness of his statement. *Of course the hospital bazaar is today, it's been advertised for the past two weeks, I've approved the newspaper ads! She must think I'm a dunce.*

Her brown eyes danced with laughter at his awkwardness. "It starts at noon." Cocking her head to the right she sized the new administrator up. "If you're executive responsibilities aren't too pressing," she said teasingly, "the hired hands could use a little help."

Wes smiled. "I've been reading old minutes of the Joint Conference Committee," he said. "Guess I could pull myself away. What do you want me to do?"

"There's two dozen cakes in the Pink Shop with no one to load them," she mused, as though trying to solve a puzzle. "And in the employee parking lot there's a hospital van with nothing in it." A faint light twinkled in her eyes. "Think you could figure something out?"

"Manual labor?" he said in mock protest. "That's not in my job description."

"It's probably more productive than anything else you've done today," she replied with an impish smile.

She was flirting with him. He didn't mind, even if the humor was at his expense. "Sounds like you've been visiting with the board about my performance," he said.

She took a breath to speak, but he interrupted by holding his hands up. "Don't comment," he said. "Just show me the way." She pointed at the Pink Shop, and then at the exit. Wes complied.

"Niels," she said turning to the custodian. "We have two more posters to hang downstairs."

"Ya. Ve better get to it," Niels said looking at his watch. Niels and Amy Castleton took the stairs to the basement.

* * *

Wes admired the luminous colors of the hillsides surrounding Park City as he drove the van to the park. The crispness of the Fall air had turned the aspen trees gold, crimson, and green. Amy and Niels followed in the hospital pick-up. When they arrived, she gave the orders, and he obeyed. He hauled cakes, refilled soft drinks, and emptied garbage cans.

The affection of the employees for Amy was obvious. Many had known her since she was an infant. Having grown up around the hospital, she returned the affection, treating the doctors and employees as family.

Amy was enthusiastic and organized, and the event was well publicized by the local newspaper and radio. In addition to the employees and medical staff, over 600 people from the community turned out for the fund raising event. There were pony rides for the kids and art exhibits for the adults. Park City's country singers, the Benton Family, provided entertainment. The bake sale raised enough money for a newborn ICU ventilator, and the five-dollar sack lunches netted funds to pay off the auto-analyzer in the lab.

For most, however, the highlight of the day was the Dunk Your Supervisor event. The Pink Ladies rented a device that dropped a chair into a large tub of water when a baseball hit the target. Employees were charged a buck a throw—members of the medical staff, three. Wes was the first to be offered the seat of honor.

Everyone cheered when Dr. Flagg hit the target, and Wes dropped into the icy water. Someone was thoughtful enough to bring dry clothes—a cotton uniform from the laundry. It was four sizes too big, so Amy fashioned a belt from a rope. Wes looked ridiculous, but was happy with the response it elicited from the employees. It broke down some of the barriers created when Wycoff fired Selman.

By late afternoon, the crowd was gone. Amy directed the cleanup. As the last car pulled out of the park, Wes loaded the sound equipment into the van. Amy climbed into the front seat with him, holding the only cake that hadn't sold. When Wes turned the key, nothing happened. He grimaced.

When he didn't move, Amy spoke. "Aren't you going to check under the hood?" she asked curiously.

"Wouldn't do any good—I don't know a carburetor from a crankshaft."

Amy studied the expression on his face, then smiled with amusement. "I take it you're not one of those macho mechanics?"

"You got it," Wes replied as he surveyed the empty parking lot.

"There's a phone at Country Corner—about four miles down the canyon. I'll walk with you!" Amy said brightly.

Wes tried the engine one more time, nothing happened. Turning to his traveling companion, he studied the cake she was holding—chocolate with green icing. The heat was turning the sliced bananas on the top an ugly brown. The bananas spelled *"Buy Me."* "What are we going to do with that?" he asked glumly.

Amy examined the gastronomic monstrosity with mock seriousness. "Do you think there's a reason it didn't sell?"

Wes nodded. "I suggest we donate it to the dumpster," he replied.

* * *

Once they were on the road and had established a consistent pace, Wes started the conversation. He had heard rumors that Amy would be returning to school.

"So what's next?" he asked.

"Mom still needs support, I'll stick around for a year"

"After that?"

"Probably return to the university."

"Do you have a major?"

"Comparative literature. Hope to teach someday." A soft canyon breeze gently stroked Amy's auburn hair. She looked at him, her eyes dancing with curiosity.

"And you, Mr. Douglas?"

"If I survive the next few months, I'll return to my accounting practice. If my administration's a disaster, then I'm not sure what I'll do, maybe pull up stakes and return to Maine."

"Is that your home?"

Wes nodded.

"Why did you leave?" she asked.

"Worked for a regional firm in Portland. Hated my supervisor, got tired of the city."

"That's all?" she asked.

Wes pondered the question, she seemed to sense that there was another reason.

"I was engaged to be married," he said quietly. "A month before our wedding, my fiancé died in an automobile accident."

"I'm sorry," she said. "How long were you engaged?"

"Three years."

"A long time."

"Too long," he said. "I was waiting until we were financially secure." His brows pulled into a brooding expression. He was silent, deep in thought and she didn't interrupt. They walked.

"There's no such thing," he said presently.

"No such thing as what?"

"Security. You can plan your life to the smallest detail, but something's always there to throw a wrench in the works."

She listened.

"When I was younger I believed there was some sort of a master plan," he continued.

"Not now?" she asked.

"It's just a game of dice."

"You sound like my mother," Amy said. "She's pretty shattered; she's become a skeptic."

"And you?" He stopped walking and they stood face to face. Her eyes reflected her gentle optimism. "I think there's a plan. It isn't ours," she continued, and usually, it's hard to see, but its there. The key, I think, is patience." She continued walking and he followed.

"Do you like your job?" she asked.

"It's interesting."

"Is that all?"

"Many of the issues are new to me."

"Have you ever worked in management before?"

"Yeah, but not in healthcare. Hospitals are a different breed of animal."

Amy raised her eyebrows in a simple question. Wes continued. "In most firms the objective is simple—maximize profit," he continued. "In hospitals, it's a little more complicated.

"How?"

"You are dealing with people's lives. The Pink Ladies just paid off the new auto-analyzer. The old one wasn't broken and it wasn't worn out. In manufacturing we don't replace equipment that still works, unless it will reduce costs or increase productivity."

"The new unit won't do either?" she asked.

"Nope."

"Then why did you buy it?"

"It does four tests the old one couldn't. We won't make any money off them, they will probably be performed less than once a month. But when we do need them, they might save a life. Financial models like *return on investment* and *internal rate of return* don't work as well in healthcare."

"Sounds like something Dad used to say," Amy said.

"Before I took this job I blamed high health care costs on inefficiency. I'm beginning to realize it's more complex than that. Take last week, for example," he continued. "Thursday I had a request from Elizabeth Flannigan that we start staffing the nursery full-time. Right now, it's monitored by the nursing station across the hall. They watch the babies through a large window."

"Our average occupancy is less than three babies a day," Wes continued. "Justifying a full-time nurse for that volume is difficult, especially when you remember we're not talking about weekdays nine to five. Full-time coverage is three shifts a day—seven days a week. It takes four full-time employees to fill one slot."

"I did the math," he said. "Full coverage would cost $126,000 a year—that's $230 for a two-day stay. There's no way I could dump that onto the nursery charge. Even if I absorb it in the overall room rate, it's still $10 a day."

"Ten dollars isn't a lot," Amy replied.

"At any time, there's a dozen legitimate proposals to increase quality," Wes countered. "Approve even the most worthy, and you increase your room rate $40 to $50 a month." His mouth spread in a thin-lipped smile. "I told them they couldn't have the coverage. Thursday afternoon," he continued, "I was on the floor and happened to look in on the Nursery. There were two newborns—twin boys, one of them was blue. I called the nurse. The baby had thrown up and aspirated. She rushed in, got him breathing again."

"Of course I stuck my head into the noose," Wes continued. "I asked her what would have happened if I hadn't come along. *He probably would have died,* she says. Then she looks at me like I'm Ebenezer Scrooge. *That's why we need full-time staffing coverage in the Nursery!* she snips.

"She was right of course. All afternoon I thought about what it would mean to have a twin brother. I could picture them playing together in preschool, venturing off arm in arm into the world on their first day of kindergarten, double-dating in high school, serving as each other's best man at their weddings. Then I contrasted that with the other scenario—the one where a young man says '*I had a twin brother, but he died several hours after we were born.*'"

Wes shrugged. "When you're faced with a situation like that, controlling costs suddenly doesn't seem very important."

16

The Model

Edward Wycoff smiled as Tony Devecchi studied the architect's model. Wycoff had commissioned it to raise capital, and it was doing its job. Jackson White, the youngest architect of Denver's most prestigious architectural firm, waited at his side, his mouth twisted tight with expectation. Two of Devecchi's business associates watched from the sidelines.

Devecchi, wearing a black shirt, white tie, and alligator shoes, circled the model like a shark examining its prey. Placing his hands on his knees, he bent over for a closer look, his small rat-like eyes greedily drinking in every detail. He swore softly, then nodded his head in approval.

"It looks different in three dimensions than it did on paper," he said, grinning broadly. "I like it! I think our young architect has done a commendable job."

Wycoff agreed. "Tell him about the project, Jackson."

Jackson took a deep breath and released it slowly. "The project will be called Wycoff Square," he said, pointing to the model. "It will consist of a hotel, condominiums, a nursing home retirement facility with three levels of care, a hospital complete with physician offices and outpatient surgery, and a shopping center."

Devecchi nodded approvingly. "Ambitious project."

"You don't make money by thinking small," an investor said.

Wycoff nodded. "It's a self-contained community. With the exception of the hotel, the project is similar to the retirement communities you've done in Arizona."

"Noticed that," Devecchi said, fishing a cigar from his shirt pocket, "but the design is better." He bit off the end of his cigar and spat it into the wastebasket. "After seeing this, I think my other projects need a new architect." With that, Devecchi nodded at Lake who beamed proudly.

"You're lucky to have such a good location," an investor commented. "Since the announcement of the Olympics, property in Park City is hard to come by."

"The project will be built on 100 acres south of Park City," Devecchi replied, turning to his associates. He pointed at the model with his cigar. "Wycoff's got the lien and assures us he'll have clear title to the property within ninety days."

"The hotel will be leased to a major hotel chain and will open before the games in 2002," Wycoff said. "Consolidated Healthcare will run the medical center. It'll be a major publicity coup for your company to be the healthcare provider for the Olympics. The advertising alone will be worth millions of dollars."

Wycoff turned to the investors. "And you gentlemen have the opportunity to provide the funding for the shopping center, provided, of course, you want to come in."

"We're in," an investor said. The others nodded. "Just see that there's no complications in getting title to the land."

A sanguine smile cracked the cold lines of Wycoff's aging face. "Gentlemen," he said with characteristic self-assurance, "it's in the bag."

✳ ✳ ✳

Wycoff was alone in the first-class section of Delta Flight 766 from Denver to Salt Lake City. He checked his watch—4:30 p.m. The Boeing 737 sat isolated at the end of runway 32, waiting a final weather check before clearance for takeoff. As Wycoff peered out his window, he noted that the day, so full of promise that morning, was fading fast as the sun closed on the lonely mountains to the west. At the airport, the temperature was dropping. Above and to the north, a pack of gray clouds hobbled across the sky, driven by an impatient westerly wind. Wycoff could feel the cold and damp in the joints of his hands.

"Ladies and gentlemen, this is the Captain speaking. We apologize for the delay. We are currently twelfth in the take-off queue."

Wycoff shrugged. *What's the hurry?* he thought. His whole life he'd been inpatient—anxious to arrive at some glorious future destination. He looked out the window at the threatening sky. *Is this all there is? A cheerless gray of old age?*

In rare moments of introspection, Wycoff reflected on the decisions of his early life. He had decided that he would avoid close personal relationships. It was a decision based on practicality—wealth and power were jealous mistresses, he wouldn't allow time for anything else. As a young man, he equated wealth and power with love and security—things he had known little of as a child. The word *surrogate* came to him. He mulled it over in his mind. Wealth was a surrogate for security and love—except it wasn't. *Counterfeit* is a better word, he reflected bitterly.

He had a wife and family, but the warmth of those relationships had died years ago, strangled by ambition that starved the affection from their marriage and choked the love from his children. He had three sons—two attorneys and a physician. A fourth child, a daughter, had taken her life at age sixteen.

The boys were polite, more out of deference to their mother than affection for their father. Their children never called him Grandfather, something he had taken pride in during their younger years.

I don't need people, Wycoff shrugged. *Friends come and go—only enemies are forever.* He was silent for a moment, then smiled sadly at his own self-deception. It was a good try. Denial worked well sometimes—today it didn't. At age seventy-nine, Edward Wycoff was concluding that there were only two tragedies in life: *Those who don't get what they truly want . . . and those who do.*

✳ ✳ ✳

Twenty minutes later Edward Wycoff gazed quietly out the window as the flight was cleared for takeoff. As the Delta 737 lifted off the runway, he reflected on how far he had come from the difficulties of his childhood.

Born the fifth son to a prosperous family, his father, Jeremiah Wycoff was a successful merchant from Rexburg, Idaho. In 1918 Jeremiah met Peter Brannan who proposed that he provide half the capital for a new bank. Although Jeremiah knew nothing about banking, the Brannans did and he invested. The Brannans at that time operated two banks, one in Park City, and a second in Price, Utah. Both were successful operations.

The bank in Rexburg prospered for six years, investing heavily in the farming community. A series of crop failures from 1925 to 1928, coupled with the Depression of 1929, severely dampened southern Idaho's economy, causing the bank to fail in 1931. Although the family blamed stress associated with the bank failure on the subsequent death of Jeremiah, they had nothing but praise for Peter Brannan. Brannan arranged for the purchase of the family's assets by a Nevada bank, including the bank stock, albeit at ten cents on the dollar.

Edward Wycoff's older sister Emily was even offered a job in the Brannan household, providing domestic help for Peter Brannan's wife, who was in failing health. Inspired by Brannan, Wycoff went east to obtain his schooling. Working his way through college, he received a degree in finance at New York University and took a job on Wall Street.

In 1933, a second tragedy struck the Wycoff family. Emily died giving birth to an illegitimate child. Edward Wycoff was told that the father, a man by the name of Raymer, had left town shortly after learning that Emily was with child. Once again, the Brannans came to the Wycoff's' rescue by arranging for the child to be raised in a home operated by the Order of Elks in Claremont, California.

Twelve years later, the fairy tale unraveled. In 1945, while researching a possible bank acquisition, Wycoff discovered that Peter Brannan had owned the Nevada bank that had purchased the Bank of Rexburg. The person the family thought was their greatest benefactor had profited from the family's financial difficulties.

Ten years later, at the deathbed of his mother, he was shocked to learn that his nephew, Ryan Raymer, was none other than the son of Peter Brannan. The Raymer story had been concocted to spare the Wycoffs and Brannans the scandal the pregnancy would have cost both families.

A rancorous palsy shook Wycoff's frame as he thought of Peter Brannan. Since that day in 1955, he had dreamed of nothing else but avenging his family. A caustic smile broke Wycoff's lips.

The chance came in 1996 while he was still on Wall Street. Word came that a small family-owned bank in Park City was up for sale. The owner, he was told, a man by the name of Brannan, had invested heavily in a software company that failed, consuming the family's fortune and placing them on the edge of bankruptcy. Further investigation revealed that other family assets, including a local newspaper could also be purchased for a small fraction of book value.

Wycoff organized a group of investors who bought the bank, the newspaper, and the mortgage. Wycoff was a silent partner—not even his wife was aware of his ownership interests in Park City.

Although the initial motivation was revenge, the announcement that Park City had obtained the 2002 Winter Olympics promised to make the transaction unbelievably profitable. The bank originally held a note on one hundred acres of land donated by the Brannans for the construction of a new hospital. The land was an ideal location for a multimillion-dollar hotel resort he and Tony Devecchi hoped to build. Although the note was paid off by the proceeds from the sale of the bank and newspaper, Wycoff knew how to get it back.

Wycoff had worked with Devecchi in the past. He was an interesting character. Originally a Philadelphia slumlord, he made most of his money through hostile takeovers. At the height of his career, he had an ownership interest in more than fifty companies. Usually, he put himself on the payroll as CEO. This provided him with annual paychecks that made him one of the highest-paid executives in the country. He then systematically looted each company through liquidation.

Wycoff knew that he would have to watch his back—he didn't trust Devecchi, but his partner had the money contacts and resources necessary to build the complex.

Wycoff's hate for the Brannan family returned, choking off any thoughts of loneliness or remorse for the way he had lived his life. For over fifty years, two goals had dominated him. The first was a desire to make money—lots of money. Money could buy security; it could buy respectability; it could buy power. The second was revenge—retribution on the family responsible for the death of his father and the disgrace of his family. With one transaction—the purchase of the Brannan estate—he was close to accomplishing both.

17

Rachel

Rachel Brannan hummed softly as she polished the teapot from the sterling silver tea set, the one her mother-in-law had given her the day she married James Brannan. She paused, holding a silver teacup to the light. The teacup was as beautiful and lustrous as the day her mother gave it to her.

Focusing on her own reflection in the cup, she smiled. Unlike the silver tea set, she had aged. The chestnut brown hair that Jim ran his fingers through the night he proposed was white, and the dark Welsh eyes he gazed into so lovingly now reflected the toils and trials of a life of hard work and service.

The more she aged, the more she reminded herself of her grandmother who had immigrated with her husband in the 1880s from the coal mines of Wales to the silver mines of Park City. Grandmother had raised her after the death of her own mother. From her grandmother, she learned the art of hard work, and hard work she did, even in her sixty-eighth year. Rachel placed the teapot on the table and studied the tea set. For thirty years, it had served as the centerpiece at the annual Governing Board and Medical Staff reception, always held at the Brannan mansion.

With Jim dead, hosting the event would be a different experience this year. She turned and gazed lovingly at his photograph on the desk. He was always good at providing direction in those areas where she was weak. Some of the family felt he provided too much direction—her son David resented his domination. For Rachel, the granddaughter of a coal miner who had never felt comfortable around rich or influential people, however, Jim's self-confidence provided comfort and security.

Rachel's thoughts were interrupted by a knock at the door. Without waiting for a response, her domestic helper Hanna Brunswick bustled into the room. Hanna carried a large linen tablecloth, which was folded over her left arm. In her right hand she held a large envelope, which she handed to Rachel. "David dropped this off this morning," she said. "You were resting. It's a list of those who've confirmed they'll be at the reception."

While Rachel opened the envelope, Hanna laid the tablecloth on the desk where Rachel could examine it. "I inventoried the linen closet this morning," she said. "This is the only one large enough to cover the serving table."

Rachel gently caressed the linen tablecloth. Like her small hand, it was frail and delicate. "The tablecloth belonged to Jim's mother. It's a shame it's getting old, but aren't we all?" she said brightly. Looking up at Hanna with brown eyes that still sparkled, she nodded. "It will be fine."

Hanna reclaimed the linen and marched out while Rachel turned her attention to the guest list. Sixty-five people would be attending in all: forty-five from the medical staff including wives, twelve from administration, and eight from the board.

My how the hospital's grown, she thought remembering the spring day in 1937 when Jim's father broke ground for the new facility in a ceremony the entire community had attended. She was only a small child, but she still remembered it. In 1937 the old Miners' Hospital was retired, and the Brannan family provided the funds for a new facility. Turning her attention back to the guest list, she scanned the names of those attending. David would be there with his wife, as would her son Matt. Matt—now *Doctor* Matt Brannan—had recently finished his internship and joined the medical staff.

At age twenty-eight, Matt was the youngest of her three children. He was sixteen years younger than her first child, a daughter who died at childbirth. For ten years after the baby's death, Rachel was continually ill, unable to conceive. Thanks to advances in gynecology, she was eventually able to have another child, David, at age thirty-five. Matt followed five years later.

Rachel took pride in the good things Matt was doing with his life. Dyslexic, Matt struggled with reading, so much so that many of their friends scoffed when Jim announced during Matt's senior year that his son wanted to become a physician. Rachel loved both of her sons, but was proudest of Matt. Now he had his education, all he needed was a wife. She smiled thoughtfully. Matt would be bringing Amy Castleton to the reception. As a member of Hap Castleton's scout troop, Matt had attained his Eagle Scout by his junior year of high school. During his college years he continued as a volunteer leader in the scout troop. Not—Rachel suspected—because he loved scouting, but because he loved Amy.

* * *

Outside, Matt Brannan was well into the annual ritual of winterizing the thirty-room mansion. The job had fallen to him as David was too impatient for the job, and their mother too old. Matt began by replacing the weather stripping on the outside doors. He was now ready to install the storm windows.

It would be best to tackle the most difficult job first, he decided, the installation of an oval storm window on the top-heavy Venetian tower. Matt shook his head as he studied the height. *It would have been nice if the great-grandfather had given some thought to energy conservation.* The original building had no insulation, and single pane windows. In 1880 coal was cheap. What's more, the builder owned the coal mines. Mike Brannan and the era in which he lived had energy to burn.

Peter Brannan, Mike's son replaced the coal furnace and had insulation blown into the attic. When the electric bill was still too high, he shopped for storm windows. Concerned that aluminum frames would distract from the architectural integrity of the building, he hired a cabinet-maker/glazier to build wooden frames, consistent in style with the arched Italianate windows. They looked nice, but were a bear to install.

With a screwdriver in one hand and pliers in the other, Matt gazed in awe at the garish old mansion. He smiled as he tried to imagine the shock on the faces of the neighbors, great-grandfather's employees, when Mike Brannan unveiled the original color scheme. Maroon walls, green trim, orange window sashes, and olive blinds.

Three stories high, the Victorian mansion with its rambling verandahs, and intricate gables, overshadowed the modest homes of the early miners. *Atypical of nineteenth century Utah—very typical of its builder,* Matt thought. *With colossal energy, ability, and enthusiasm, great-grandfather was bigger than life. So was his house.*

Standing in the shadow of the old mansion, Matt felt small and inconsequential. Old feelings of inadequacy returned. Heir apparent to the Brannan legacy, Matt had inherited his great-grandfather's appearance, but little of his genius or energy. Eyes wide with apprehension, Matt Brannan placed a tall ladder against the family icon, then carefully climbed the ornate façade of the three-story tower.

18

The Plan Takes Shape

Saturday evening, Rachel Brannan hosted the yearly medical staff reception. Wes Douglas used the opportunity to learn more about the medical staff's perceptions of Peter Brannan Community Hospital. Many were concerned about the vacuum created by Hap's death. The medical staff feared that Wycoff would use this void to push his cost-cutting agenda even further.

Dr. Emil Flagg bent Wes's ear on the dangers of corporate medicine. For thirty minutes, he extolled the virtues of a hospital administrator who was unwilling to subject the medical staff to the "dual degradation of budgeting and managed care." Flagg was especially critical of HMOs that controlled patient flows.

"Some of our doctors have spent twenty years building their medical practices," he said. "They aren't worth a nickel now. HMOs own their patients."

"The older docs feel betrayed," he continued, "disconnected from the healthcare system they helped build. The people who run HMOs are nothing more than bookies. They hire statisticians to study the probabilities of morbidity and mortality, then figure out ways to keep all the profits by shifting the risk to the doctors and the hospitals."

Dr. Amos took a more moderate view. "I agree with what Krimmel says about the need for a market mechanism. The old system wasn't good at involving all the stakeholders, but managed care isn't solving the problem either. We're substituting efficiency for thoroughness and quality. That's a scary trade-off when you're dealing with human lives."

"Since insurance companies are paying the bill, they're dictating practice protocols, a domain that belongs exclusively to physicians. Managed care is becoming another bureaucracy. Only this time it's sponsored by the private sector rather than by government."

The evening brought other revelations. Amy Castleton accompanied Dr. Matt Brannan. Wes noticed how he worshipfully followed her around as she visited with the physicians and their wives. He was developing a deep visceral dislike for Matt. He couldn't identify a specific reason, or at least not one he was willing to admit it to himself.

* * *

Monday afternoon, Wes met with Natalie Simpson to develop a plan that would put the hospital at breakeven within ninety days of the date the bank had renewed the hospital's line of credit. "Hospitals lose money by generating too little revenue or incurring too much cost," Wes said. "Let's focus on costs first."

Natalie brought comparative productivity and cost information from the Utah Healthcare Association to the meeting. Of special interest were comparative data on average cost per patient day for labor and materials for hospitals approximately the same size as Peter Brannan Community Hospital. The data clearly showed that PBCH had higher costs than any other primary-care hospital in its size category in the state. For the next two hours, Wes analyzed the data in an attempt to understand why.

As a manufacturing consultant, Wes relied on standard cost accounting systems that provided cost variances on production. A *variance* is the difference between what a product *should cost* and what it *actually costs.* Variances help managers *understand the reasons* for cost overruns. Wes knew that the two most common reasons for an unfavorable labor or material variance are (1) the company paid too much for the resource or (2) the company used too much of the resource.

The manufacturing industry had been using standard cost accounting since the late nineteenth century. It was a relatively new development in healthcare, however, although a number of hospitals had installed some form of standard costing since the advent of prospective payment.

Establishing a standard costing system at Peter Brannan Community Hospital was one of Wes's primary objectives. Since labor consumed 30 percent of his hospital's total budget, he decided to focus on labor standards first.

That afternoon, Wes called Karisa Holyoak. She gave him the name of Dr. Irene Cowdrey, a professor of management at Weber State University who had helped some of Holyoak's clients establish fair and competitive labor rates. This would be the first step in designing a standard cost accounting system.[2] A meeting with Cowdrey and Don Yanamura (the hospital's human resource director) was established for the following day.

✴ ✴ ✴

"Your problem is similar to that of a number of other clients of mine," said Irene Cowdrey. Cowdrey was a fifty-year-old college professor who consulted regularly in compensation.

"Your compensation system was developed over a number of years on an ad-hoc basis as the hospital added new positions," she continued. "There were no guidelines— no governing philosophies. As a result, your salary schedules lack *internal consistency* and *external validity.*"

"What does that mean?" Yanamura asked.

"Internal consistency means that the system is *fair—employees get equal pay for equal work.* External validity means that a firm's salaries are *consistent with the market.* Utah Healthcare Association data indicate your salaries are neither."

Yanamura gave Wes a side-glance. "I suspected that was the case," he said. "I inherited the present system. I've never had the resources to fix it."

---

[2] Standard costing determines variances. To calculate a labor variance, Wes will need four pieces of information: (1) the standard labor rate, (2) the standard labor quantity, (3) the actual labor rate, and (4) the actual labor quantity. Irene Cowdrey's study will provide a methodology to establish the standard labor rate.

Cowdrey smiled sympathetically. "That's a problem many personnel directors face," she said. "They're often so busy with daily operations they don't have time to design proper systems."

"I'd think most hospitals would be ripe for the service you offer," Yanamura said.

"That's true. Technology keeps changing the content of hospital jobs, and that creates problems with compensation, recruitment, training, and performance evaluation."

Wes was pleased that Yanamura was receptive. "If we hire your firm, how long would it take you to design a market-based compensation system for the hospital?" he asked. "A system that would provide standard labor cost for a new cost accounting system?"

Cowdrey retrieved a calculator from her briefcase and punched in several figures. "You have about two hundred employees—about 125 different job descriptions," she said. "My firm completed a similar project for Memorial Hospital in Colorado Springs. I think we could finish your study in about six weeks."

Yanamura nodded at Wes, who turned to Cowdrey. "I wish we could get the data faster, but if six weeks is your best estimate, that'll have to do. Keep me posted on your progress."

* * *

For a discussion on the use of multiple regression to establish standard labor rates see Supplement Two, "Variance Analysis," which is found in the appendix. This is recommended reading for all students who plan to hold a supervisory or administrative position in healthcare.

* * *

For a more detailed discussion of variance analysis and cost roll-ups, See Supplement Three, "Calculating Labor Variances." This is recommended reading for health administration and accounting students.

19

Inadequately Trained

Except for Dr. Matt Brannan, the medical library was empty. At a table in the far corner he quietly read the medical record of a former patient. His eyes were wide with disbelief as he examined the lateral x-ray. *How could I miss that?* Small beads of perspiration formed on his upper lip as he re-read the notes of Dr. Frank Almond, an emergency room physician who had seen the toddler four hours after Dr. Brannan sent her home.

In Brannan's pocket was a letter from the Mortality and Morbidity Committee, a peer review group with the charter to identify substandard practice on the medical staff. The letter requested that he come to a breakfast meeting the following Monday, prepared to discuss the case of Brittany Anderson. The letter charged that he had misdiagnosed her case, with almost fatal consequence.

A week ago a young mother, Jonel Anderson had brought her three-year-old daughter Brittany to his office. The initial examination revealed a barking cough and a mildly elevated temperature of 101.1 degrees. The child was drooling, a sign Brannan should have paid more attention to but didn't—*toddlers drool*, he reasoned. Brittany's breathing was labored, which he mis-attributed to congestion or a stuffed up nose.

The lab work was normal, except for a slightly elevated white blood count of eleven. To rule out pneumonia Brannan ordered a chest x-ray, AP (anterior posterior) and lateral views. He should have checked for epiglotitis but didn't.

Since her lungs were clean, he concluded that she had a case of viral, upper respiratory track infection (URI). He sent her home. "There's nothing we can do for her in the hospital that you can't do at home," he told the worried mother. "Give her plenty of fluids, monitor temperature, give her Tylenol if her temperature increases, and call me if it gets worse."

Three hours later, cyanotic, and in acute respiratory arrest, Britanny Anderson was brought to the Emergency Room by ambulance. Her epiglottis, now severely swollen, had sealed off her airway. So severe was the swelling, that it was almost impossible to intubate her. Brittany Anderson almost died in the hospital's emergency room.

In today's review of Britanny's records, he saw now what he missed earlier, the characteristic thumb print sign on the lateral x-ray—a sure indicator of acute epiglotitis. Dr. Brannan finished reading and closed the medical record. This would be the second time in a year that he would be called before the committee. He was fearful they would conclude what he himself suspected, that he was inadequately trained to practice family medicine.

Dr. Brannan was tired of feelings of inadequacy, thoughts he experienced since his father first made the decision that Matt would go into medicine. The Brannan family had an image in the community that was larger than life. Only medicine would be an acceptable career for the youngest heir to the Brannan legacy.

Matt explained to his father that he was a slow reader and not a good student. No matter, James enrolled him in the university and hired the best tutors money could buy. Hard study, good tutoring, and a family endowment of one million dollars to a small medical college on the east coast assured Matt's acceptance to the class of 1994.

It wasn't easy, but Matt hung in there. Four years later, he graduated, ninety-fifth in a class of 103 students. He completed a one-year internship and was applying for a residency in family practice when the family's fortune started to disintegrate, his father had a stroke, and Matt was called home to help put the family back together. As always, the family's needs came first. The residency would have to wait.

The library was quiet except for the ticking of a large grandfather clock on the far wall. Matt's mother had presented it to the medical staff in appreciation for the care Jim had received after his stroke. Dr. Brannan's eyes narrowed, and deep lines of determination formed around his mouth. *I need more training.*

Reviewing his options, he stared at a bookshelf on the far wall. On the second shelf was a directory that listed family practice residencies in the United States. He would apply for a residency, if that wasn't good enough, he would follow it with a fellowship. The only complication was Amy Castleton. He had given his heart completely; she had yet to do the same. They had discussed marriage. She had not accepted his many proposals and was now dating others, among them Wes Douglas. If Matt went back to school without her, he was sure that she wouldn't be here when he returned.

✳ ✳ ✳

"Knock, knock," Helen Castleton said as she slowly opened the door to Amy's bedroom.

Amy, sitting at her vanity by the window looked up and blinked brightly. "What do you think of the makeup?" she asked. "It's a new color."

"Absolutely stunning." Carrying a black dress, Mrs. Castleton crossed the room to Amy's closet. "Picked this up from the cleaners. Thought you might like to wear it tonight. It's one of Matt's favorites, isn't it?"

Amy nodded. "I'm not going out with Matt tonight," she said, returning to the mirror. "The film festival's in town, and Wes Douglas has asked me to go with him."

Helen's eyes registered her surprise. "Wes Douglas?" she said. "The new administrator?"

Amy nodded. Her mother was silent as she processed Amy's message. Finally she spoke, choosing her words carefully. "I don't think things are going well for him at the hospital," she said. "In some ways I wonder if it's a good idea for you to date him."

"Why?"

"He has a financial background, some think he's a miniature Edward Wycoff. There are those who think he wants to change things from the way they were under your father—to run the hospital more like a business, not a charity."

Amy shrugged. "That might not be all bad, given their current situation with the bank."

Helen shot Amy a withering look. "Your father would turn over in his grave if he thought you were siding with the accountants. You remember the fights he had with Wycoff?"

"I'm not siding with Wycoff," Amy said wearily. "It just seems like times have changed and—"

"The doctors don't like what's going on," Helen continued. "They're unhappy the board didn't consult them before appointing Mr. Douglas as interim administrator. There's talk of a revolt."

Amy began brushing her hair. "Where'd you hear that, Mom?"

"Rachel Brannan," Helen replied. "She thinks they should appoint Matt as interim administrator."

Amy smiled. "I'm sure she's a competent judge," She replaced the brush on the dresser. Finished, she shook her head until her hair fell softly on her shoulders. Amy stood and retrieved her dress from the closet.

"Rachel says Matt's got a lot of good ideas on how to run the hospital. Maybe they'd put him in permanently."

"Anybody ask Matt what he thinks of the idea?" Amy asked.

Rachel thinks he'd make a fine administrator, and so do I. He certainly would carry on the tradition of the family."

"Whose family—ours or theirs?" Amy asked dryly.

"Well, maybe both," Helen replied. "I thought you and Matt were talking of marriage."

"Matt's talking; I'm listening."

"You do love him?" Helen asked, her eyes reflecting her curiosity.

"Yes, I do, Mom," Amy sighed. "At least I think I do. It's just that I've known him since I was six, and sometimes it seems—"

"I think Rachel has her heart set on a Christmas engagement," Helen said.

"Well, I'm not engaged yet," Amy said as she slipped into her dress. Cocking her head slightly, she smiled. "I think that's the doorbell, Mom."

Helen gave her a resigned smile. Amy had her father's stubbornness as well as his charm. "I can see I'm not going to change your mind tonight," she said. "I'll get the door."

Amy shot her a look of warning.

"Okay, I'll even be nice," Helen said.

* * *

Actor Robert Redford started the Sundance Film Festival in 1981, hoping to create an event that would support independent filmmaking. Through the years it grew, attaining international stature. In 1999, over three hundred young filmmakers showcased their work before many of Hollywood's most talented producers, writers, and actors. Each year the public is invited.

On the evening of their first date, Wes Douglas and Amy Castleton saw two films and later dined at the Olive Barrel Food Company, a small restaurant on Main Street. "I met your mother at the medical staff reception at the Brannans," Wes began while they were waiting for their order.

"It was difficult for her to go without Dad."

"You were there with Matt Brannan," Wes said, watching the expression on her face. He was interested in knowing more about their relationship. "How long have you known each other?"

"Our families have been close for many years. Father, of course, worked closely with Matt's father on the board."

Wes nodded, and waited for her to continue.

"Rachel and I are close. Before we moved to Park City, she and Jim lost a baby girl. Maybe I helped fill a void. I spent a lot of time in the Brannan household when I was growing up. It was only natural that Matt and I would become friends. Dad liked Jim Brannan; they were both good fishermen. Jim Brannan had a cabin on the Salmon River."

"Hap had a lot of friends," Wes said.

"He got energy from people," Amy acknowledged, "and he is was good to everyone. It was interesting to see the diversity of people that turned out for his funeral. Everyone from the governor to the humblest housekeeper were there, he had always treated them the same. I think everyone there considered themselves a close friend of Hap Castleton."

"One of his pallbearers spent some time with me after the service," Amy continued. "A fellow by the name of Arthur Skyros. Dad met him when Art's mother Marie moved to Park City in 1985, three weeks after her husband was imprisoned for holding up a liquor store in Los Angeles. Marie got a job in the hospital laundry. I think that the transition from Los Angeles to Park City was difficult for Art. He was poorer than most of the kids at the high school. He looked different and talked different—and eventually, of course, the word got out about his father."

"Dad became aware of the situation when Marie left work one day to bail Art out of jail for shoplifting. That evening, Dad showed up at the basement room Marie had rented to invite Art to join his scout troop. Marie hesitated. Dad suspected it was because they didn't have the money for a scout uniform. Dad retrieved one from a former scout, and took him to the next meeting."

"Some scouts looked down their noses at Art—his father wasn't a physician or an attorney. Dad was pretty tough and never allowed down-talk. Eventually Art was accepted by the other boys and became one of Hap's best scouts. When Art graduated from high school, Dad used the fact that Art had obtained the rank of Eagle Scout to get a former hospital trustee to fund a scholarship for him."

"Art worked hard in college. Four years later, Dad was the second person he called when he received his letter of acceptance to medical school. Art is now in his third year and wants to specialize in pediatrics."

"Shortly after Art joined the scout troop, Dad got the family out of their basement apartment. The hospital owned several homes adjacent to the physician's parking lot. They were purchased for future expansion. One of these he rented to Marie for $150 a month. When her arthritis became so bad she could no longer work, he lowered the rent to $50.

"One day while reviewing the books, Edward Wycoff found out about it. The small house could have been rented out for twenty times that amount during ski season. He hit the ceiling and wanted Dad censured for misusing hospital assets. Dad offered to retroactively pay the difference. The board heard him out, then ruled that wasn't necessary. Marie had been a faithful employee for many years, and she stayed in the home. Not everyone on the board was as bottom-line oriented as Edward Wycoff."

"Dad may not have been the best businessman in the world," Amy continued, "but his heart was in the right place. He was intensely loyal to his employees, and most of them loved him for it."

"That's a tribute to your father," Wes said. He was beginning to understand the motive for many of the things Hap Castleton had done during his tenure as administrator of Peter Brannan Community Hospital. It was interesting to contrast the value systems of Hap Castleton and Edward Wycoff. Wycoff had made millions, Hap had died with few material assets. *I'm not sure I am willing to judge who was the most successful,* Wes thought.

* * *

From deep inside the down comforter, Amy Castleton arched her back lazily. Curling her toes, she rubbed her legs against the soft flannel sheets, comfortably warm in the cold morning air of her attic bedroom. Sighing comfortably, she rolled onto her back, stretching her arms high above her head. It was Saturday morning. As she stirred, she gently pulled the covers from her head.

Sitting up, she hugged her knees, blissfully happy, but not sure why. She suspected Wes Douglas had something to do with it. The morning sunlight flowed from the compass window above her bed, giving the room an ethereal glow. The bedroom smelled of potpourri and cedar. Situated on the second floor, the bedroom windows were level with the maple trees that bordered Grand Avenue.

As a little girl, her bedroom was her castle tower—a place to wait for her prince. This morning, the same magic hung in the air. Had he come? Tilting her head, she lazily turned the idea over in her mind. She settled back into the bed as her eyes traced the sculpture of the heavy ceiling beams. Hap Castleton carved them himself from Cedar he hauled from southern Utah. She smiled as she remembered how her father loved working with wood. To Hap, there was something sacred about that medium. "Wood shouldn't be forced out," he said, "but shaped and fitted together like an interlocking puzzle." Dad took the same approach with people.

Hap built the home their first year in Park City. Carpentry served as an emotional outlet as Hap struggled to retool himself from a building contractor into a healthcare executive. The job change wasn't easy. He wouldn't have attempted it, but for the encouragement of Jim Brannan, the first to see Hap's managerial potential.

Hap, a contractor in Southern California, built a summer home for the Brannans in the foothills above Glendale, California. Brannan appreciated his honesty and work ethic—but, most of all, his ability to work well with subcontractors of different backgrounds, temperaments, and personalities. Peter Brannan Community Hospital's former administrator had announced his retirement, and Jim Brannan had his eye out for a replacement.

Park City was still transitioning from a primitive mining town to a sophisticated ski resort. Its struggling hospital needed someone who could pull the ethnically and culturally diverse community together. Not long after Brannan's summer home was finished, interest rates went through the ceiling, and Castleton's construction business folded. Brannan hired Hap to manage the hospital.

The move from Glendale, California, to Park City was easy for Hap—but not for his wife. She wanted a home. It was not easy for a man who had filed bankruptcy to obtain a construction loan. With a little arm-twisting by Jim Brannan, however, the bank loaned the funds for the materials and Hap provided the labor.

Hap built the home of stone, brick, and redwood. It had the architectural elements of a California bungalow. With broad latticed eaves, open porches, and expressive uses of wood, an article in the *Park City Herald* called it "Japanesque." Whatever its style, the gabled, trellised, and shingled home reflected Hap's personality—functional, friendly, masculine, but, most of all, unique.

Sitting up now, Amy basked in the ambience of the room. She had many happy memories in this place—tea parties in kindergarten, sleepovers in junior high, prepping for dates with Matt Brannan in high school.

Her eyes narrowed thoughtfully as she considered Matt. He had been a part of her life from their first day in Park City. Initially he filled the role of an older brother. Later she learned that his feelings were deeper. Three years older than she, he followed her through high school with worshipful awe, careful to do nothing that would frighten her away while he waited for her to grow up. He was always kind, always there. The relationship grew, and so did her feelings for him.

It was an effortless relationship—secure but not very exciting. Did she love him? Or was she merely comfortable? With dating, school and volunteer work, her life had settled into a dependable routine, shattered now by her father's accident.

Amy musingly cocked her head. *And now there's Mr. Wes Douglas—am I falling for him?* She wasn't sure. Wes was different than Matt Brannan. Amy dominated the relationship with Matt. She led and Matt followed. Stronger, more deliberate, Wes Douglas stirred her feelings. Her forehead furrowed into a deep scowl. The whole thing was unsettling.

* * *

The return address was The Department of Justice in Denver, Colorado. Sensing its importance, the controller's secretary pulled the official looking envelope from the stack of department mail and placed it prominently on Natalie Simpson's desk where she would be sure to see it upon returning from lunch.

In a few minutes, the young controller returned. Her secretary was right, it was important! Picking it up, she crossed the office and shut the door. Returning to her desk she opened the envelope, fingers trembling. She hoped her fears would be put to rest, she had a propensity to worry, and most of the things she worried about never happened. *Only, why had the Department of Justice waited so long to issue its report?* Carefully unfolding the document, she scanned the introductory letter, her pupils narrowing as she searched for key words.

She gasped in sudden surprise. *No—it couldn't be right, she must be missing something. Maybe she read it too fast.* More slowly now, she read the letter from the beginning, then read it again.

Two years ago, the hospital received its first letter from the Department of Justice requesting information on the hospital's billing methods. Eight months later, after spending $30,000 on audit fees, Natalie submitted seven years' worth of information. Sixteen months passed, and the hospital heard nothing. Now a letter informed them that they owed $749,532, not for fraud, but for an infringement of rules. The hospital had followed a long-standing practice of billing for laboratory tests one at a time. Medicare wanted them bundled.

This was the second infringement in a three-month period. Earlier, the hospital received a demand for the return of $1,200,000 in Medicare payments for radiology services provided over a three-year period. The government claimed the hospital used the wrong billing code. Although the difference in revenue between the two codes was only $125,000, the Feds wanted *all* the money back. They claimed that the deadline for rebilling under the correct code had passed.

The Federal Government was in trouble with healthcare spending and was determined to cut costs—by hook or crook. The number of FBI agents assigned to Medicare fraud had been dramatically increased. *"It's almost a manhunt,"* an article in *Forbes Magazine* that Natalie had read reported. *"With that many cops out there, they've got to justify their keep. More and more, simple mistakes and misunderstandings are being labeled as fraud."*

The article quoted J. D. Klenke, a prominent medical economist: *"The whole focus on infringement, as opposed to flagrant violation, means everybody's guilty. There are 45,000 pages of Medicare reimbursement regulations. If you violate something on page 44,391—you're guilty. Full compliance is not possible. The regulations are Byzantine."*

Some larger hospitals in the state had hired in-house compliance officers whose sole job was to read rules and regulations. Given the tight budget, Natalie had resisted increasing her staff. *Obviously a mistake, given the Justice Department ruling and the legal cost the hospital would incur to fight it.*

Natalie wasn't opposed to going after the bad guys. With national expenditures for healthcare exceeding a trillion dollars a year, there was bound to be fraud. What she objected to, however, was a federal agency whose goal was revenue, not law enforcement. She shook his head as she laid the letter on his desk. *Hospital accounting wasn't fun anymore.*

20

Raymer

"Take two tablets twice a day—on an empty stomach," groused Ryan Raymer, chief pharmacist, as he handed a prescription to the last customer of the day. It was 6:30, and his feet ached. He'd have been out of this prison if it weren't for the babbling of eighty-two-year-old Zola Wayment, a retired hospital employee who frequented the pharmacy with minor complaints and stupid questions.

Zola held the bottle close to her face as she slowly read the label. Raymer drummed his fingers on the white Formica counter, his lips drawn tight with impatience. Satisfied that the pharmacist had filled the prescription correctly, Zola carefully placed the bottle in her purse, retrieved a $20 bill, and handed it to him.

Without a reply, he grabbed it, shoved the change across the counter, and slammed shut the metal security window that separated the pharmacy from the hall. Most evenings, the end of the shift would have been a time for rejoicing. He was never meant for the drudgery of shift work. Tonight, however, things were different. In nine hours, he would be meeting with Barry Zaugg, a two-bit drug runner for Sid Carnavali, the main distributor for the drug lab he had established two months ago. It wasn't Zaugg he worried about. He didn't have the IQ to lace his shoes. Zaugg's boss, however, was a different matter. Carnavali was capable of murder.

A wave of apprehension swept over Raymer. He removed a handkerchief and wiped the beads of sweat from his brow. He had problems—big problems—and Carnavali could make them worse. As he began the nightly task of balancing the cash register, his stomach churned. He reflected on the course that had brought him to this frightening juncture in his life.

Money was the problem—and always had been—since he'd married Betty. The daughter of a successful physician, Betty had been raised to expect a lifestyle that Raymer couldn't provide. She never let him forget it. At first, he made up the difference between his income and her expenditures by taking money from the till. It was a slick routine.

Each evening after closing, he would destroy the master tape from the cash register, then re-ring the day's transactions. The new total would always be $200 or so less than the day's actual revenue—money he would pocket before leaving for home. The hospital had sloppy financial controls, his need was great, and the opportunity was there.

Over a three-year period, Raymer embezzled approximately $180,000 from the hospital. He'd have gotten a lot more, but an accounting student from Weber State University serving an internship in the Business Office had noticed that transaction numbers on the master tape didn't correspond to those shown on customer receipts.

Raymer fired the student, claiming he made a pass at a high school girl who worked part time in the pharmacy.

Raymer quit re-ringing the register. When financial pressures reappeared, he started moonlighting evenings at a local nursing home, filling prescriptions for patients from the extended care center's in-house pharmacy. At Raymer's suggestion, the nursing home began purchasing its drugs through the hospital. Hap Castleton approved of the practice because it provided the volume necessary for volume discounts for both medical facilities.

One evening, a fire destroyed the nursing home's kitchen and adjoining pharmacy. Raymer didn't know how it started, but he took advantage of it. Returning to the hospital that evening, he filled a predated nursing home order for $6,000 of narcotics, which he removed from the hospital and sold to a drug dealer named Carnavali. The drugs, which netted $18,000 on the street, he reported as having been delivered to the nursing home, prior to the fire.

It was a good trick, but it couldn't be replicated. He couldn't go around burning down nursing homes. One of the residents of the nursing home, however, was a retired physician in early stages of mental dementia. With funding from Carnavali, Raymer established a bogus home health agency in Salt Lake City, using the physician's narcotics number to write prescriptions, which he sold to Carnavali. The practice ended six months later when the physician died from old age.

Financial pressure returned when Raymer's son, Ronnie, announced shortly after high school graduation that he wanted to attend the same private university that Betty had attended. Raymer had heard of a group of pharmacists in Sweden who had been caught making street drugs from over-the-counter medications. With his knowledge as a pharmacist and with help from the *Pharmacopedia*, Raymer was soon able to duplicate the Swedish process.

His brother-in-law, Hank Ulman, owned part interest in a small flight service that operated out of the Salt Lake Airport. Business was slow, so Raymer helped him get a job to supplement his income in hospital maintenance. The plan was to have Hank fly the drugs to Phoenix. Carnavali would handle the marketing.

One obstacle was the large quantities of over-the-counter medications that would have to be purchased as raw materials for the process. Large purchase orders from local distributors tipped off the authorities in Sweden. Raymer solved the problem by purchasing the medications through the hospital and running them through the books of his home health agency. To avoid having to remove the bulky raw materials from the hospital for processing, Raymer established a small lab in a room beneath the pharmacy storeroom. It was a sweet setup.

Raymer's business was threatened, however, when Roger Selman hired a new assistant by the name of Del Cluff. Del, a former auditor, became suspicious. Curious as to why a home health agency would buy so many over-the-counter drugs, he requested copies of all purchase orders from the home health agency. Raymer could have handled the problem, but Carnavali panicked.

The evening before Cluff had been scheduled to fly with Castleton to Idaho, Carnavali paid Ulman to silence Cluff by sabotaging the plane. Hap stored his plane in a hangar near Ulman's flight service. Castleton was killed, but Cluff survived, albeit in a coma at University Hospital.

Shortly after the accident, Ulman broke into Cluff's office and stole his audit work papers. A permanent solution to the Cluff problem was yet to be reached.

The cash register balanced. Raymer removed the day's receipts, depositing them in a small safe in his office. Finished with the day's activities, he turned the lights off, locked the pharmacy, and headed for the employee parking lot. In nine hours he would be back—this time to meet with Zaugg.

✱ ✱ ✱

"Get in here before somebody sees you," Raymer whispered as he pulled Barry Zaugg through the pharmacy door.

Zaugg swore. "It's three in the morning!" he protested, twisting free from Raymer's grip. "This place is abandoned." He rubbed his arm and then slugged Raymer in the same place. "And keep your wretched hands off me!"

Raymer winced. "Hospitals are never abandoned," he warned as he shut the door. "Follow me." Crossing the room, Raymer fished in his pocket for his keys and then unlocked a door to the adjacent storeroom. Zaugg followed him through the door. A naked light bulb on the ceiling lit the bile green walls. An abandoned desk, filthy with dust, stood next to a yellowed 1971 calendar. Empty cabinets covered an adjacent wall.

"Used to be the administrator's office," Raymer said, kicking his way through the boxes that littered the black and red linoleum floor. "When the administrative wing was added in 1972, the pharmacy took it over as a storeroom. "Don't use it for much anymore," he continued, "but it makes a good cover for the lab. That's why I always keep it locked," he said, waving his key.

"I don't see no lab," Zaugg said.

Raymer stopped and rested his right hand on a wooden storage shelf. "Used to be a door here," he said. "When my brother-in-law started work here, I had him build this cabinet. "It swings out," he said, "but you have to unlock it of course."

Raymer scowled as he searched for the right key on his chain. "Here it is," he said, bending over and inserting the key into a lock on the underside of the bottom shelf. There was a metallic click. Raymer removed the key and the cabinet swung open, revealing a small stairwell.

"They kept the safe down here," he said, entering the stairwell. He flipped a light switch. "Don't think anybody knows about it anymore." Raymer continued down the stairs, Zaugg following close behind. "All the old employees have retired, and I don't let any of the new ones into the storeroom."

At the bottom of the stairs, Raymer turned on another light. "Hank works in the shop. Got hold of the original hospital blueprints, the ones the carpenters use for remodeling. He redrew the wall so the stairwell doesn't show. On the master blueprint, it looks like the pharmacy on the other side is three feet wider at this point than it actually is."

Zaugg followed him through the door, then stopped. Lighting a cigarette, he inhaled deeply, letting the acrid smoke trickle out of his nose as he surveyed the room. Roughly fifteen feet square, its concrete walls were bare, damp, and sour. A single frayed electrical cord dangled from the ceiling like a hangman's noose, its mustard light giving Zaugg's face a cadaver-like appearance. In the center sat an old autopsy table from pathology, cluttered with beakers, bottles, and a Bunsen burner.

"This is it?" Zaugg asked, gesturing with his cigarette. "This is the meth lab?"

"It's all it takes," Raymer replied, his eyes glowing with pride. "Took me a couple of weeks to figure out how it's done, another month to figure out how to get the raw materials without arousing suspicion. I've run two test samples, and now I'm ready for production."

Zaugg nodded slowly. "Good thing," he said. "It's been two months since Carnavali paid you. Thirty thousand bucks. The boys in Phoenix are getting anxious for their delivery."

"You've seen the lab." Raymer blinked defensively. "Tell them they'll get their first shipment a week from Friday. I leave Friday for Connecticut. I'll be gone three days—I'm visiting my boy in college." Raymer removed a picture of his son and proudly placed it on the table. "His name's Ronny. He wants to go to medical school."

Raymer wasn't sure why it was important to impress this thug. Maybe it was to let him know that he wasn't a common crook, like Carnavali. "When I return Monday night," he continued, "I go to work. Figure in four days I'll have the first shipment—it'll pay off Carnavali and then some."

A cold silence engulfed him as Zaugg nodded slowly. "Hope so," he said. Raymer noticed Zaugg's cold gray eyes were the color of death as he crushed his cigarette out on the boy's picture. "Carnavali don't have no patience for deadbeats. No patience at all," he said.

21

Direct Materials

Monday morning, Wes turned his attention to data from the Utah Healthcare Association that showed that Peter Brannan Community Hospital had a higher-than-average cost of materials per patient day. For the next two days, he reviewed the materials function with Anne Leavitt, director of materials management. At their concluding meeting, he summarized the following problems:

- The hospital is not participating in the Utah Healthcare Association's group purchasing contracts. Consequently, it is paying more for medical supplies than most of its competitors.

- The hospital has a large number of open purchase orders with local vendors. Authority to purchase is not clearly identified. Misuse of purchasing authorization is possible.

- The hospital has never considered a just-in-time material management system. Just-in-time is feasible as many of Peter Brannan Community Hospital's vendors have warehouses in Salt Lake City.

- There are no economic order quantities. Some nursing stations have excessive levels of inventory, as nurses are fearful of running out of supplies when Central Supply is closed on weekends and in the evenings.

Having received little direction from Hap, Anne was receptive to the new administrator's suggestions. Together, they prepared a plan to address these problems. Wes presented the plan to Natalie Simpson the following morning.

Natalie agreed with Wes's ideas and suggested that as he was investigating the hospital's purchasing practices, that he look into the practices of the pharmacy as well. It was her observation that Ryan Raymer had a lifestyle that exceeded his income. Natalie reported the pharmacy lacked defined purchasing procedures and didn't make nightly deposits. This led to a discussion of other questionable practices that Hap had never allowed Natalie to address.

In May, for example, an audit revealed that the hospital's maintenance supervisor had built a fence at his home with materials acquired on a hospital purchase order. Reimbursement had never been made. Castleton was reticent to fire the supervisor, as he had been at the hospital for twenty-five years and was two weeks away from an honorable retirement.

Natalie suspected that the business office manager had an ownership interest in the agency used by the hospital to collect bad debts, an obvious conflict of interest as the business office manager was the one responsible for determining which accounts were given to the collection agency.

At the conclusion of their meeting, Wes asked that Natalie conduct internal audits on the pharmacy, on Maintenance, and on the Business Office. Wes hoped that audit findings would be negative and that the firing of dishonest employees would not be necessary. If employee terminations were required, however, Wes planned to make them as soon as possible. *Move quickly and take no hostages,* he decided.

* * *

Fridays were slow days for the Pink Shop. Except for emergency procedures, the operating room was closed and the census was down. Fewer patients meant fewer visitors and, therefore, fewer Pink Shop customers. Amy Castleton served as the secretary/treasurer of the women's volunteer organization. Fridays were a good time to work on the books. Today, Amy's goal was to reconcile the bank statements. For the third time in an hour, she picked up the August statement and then laid it back on the counter.

Her mind wouldn't focus. The problem was Matt Brannan. Somehow, Matt had gotten word that Amy was still dating the new administrator, and he was livid.

"He's a CPA for heaven sakes," Matt's tone was accusatory, as though Amy were somehow to blame for his vocation. "He is cut from the same mold as Edward Wycoff. Profits are the only thing he worries about; patients are means to an end, they're nothing more than work-in-process."

From her own work in the Pink Shop, Amy understood the importance of not running in the red. Given the financial condition of the hospital, she appreciated the problems the hospital's losses were causing for Wes. How to solve these problems was a primary source of contention between the board and the medical staff.

Prior to his death, Hap told her the board favored a managed care approach. He explained, "Managed care seeks to control hospital costs through more efficient utilization of resources. Some of the ways it does this are peer reviews, pre-certification, financial incentives to encourage physicians to use fewer services, and the use of gatekeeper physicians to assure that expensive specialists are only used when needed."

Managed care troubled Hap. Insurance company clerks who did not have the medical background necessary to question physician decisions performed utilization review. On a daily basis, insurance companies challenged physicians with questions like *"Is this procedure experimental?"* or *"Is there a less expensive medication or procedure that can be used?"*

"Medicine has always been *experimental,"* Hap said. "That's why they call it the *practice of medicine.* To refuse to pay for a procedure that hasn't been tried in the past is to close the door on innovation and future research. There are diagnostic procedures that are less expensive than CAT scans, but these are invasive, more painful, and often more dangerous to the patient. Specialists *are* more expensive than general practitioners," Hap continued, "but that's because they know more. Since when do we want to *'dumb down'* medicine?"

As for incentive reimbursement, Hap recognized the problems with traditional fee-for-service and cost reimbursement but was not convinced that forcing physicians to select treatment options based on cost rather than quality was the right approach.

To illustrate the point, he showed Amy a note an internist had received on an order for a CAT scan. The procedure was for a patient whom the physician feared had a brain tumor. *"Approve this, and it will be your last,"* a handwritten note on the letter said. In the same envelope, the physician received a list of the insurance company's participating physicians, sorted by cost per patient per diagnosis. The physician's name was on the top third of the list. *"Expensive providers will be eliminated from participation in our physician panels unless they change practice patterns,"* a note attached to the list explained.

Amy's father had been hesitant to embrace managed care—until he could be assured that quality would not suffer. Wycoff believed that Hap's reticence brought the hospital to the brink of insolvency. The medical staff believed that Wycoff's approach would destroy the purpose for which hospitals were formed in the first place—*to provide the highest quality of care to patients, regardless of their ability to pay.*

Matt was certain that Wes Douglas was evolving into a young Edward Wycoff. He accused Wes of using Amy's father as the fall guy for the hospital's current financial situation. "He's slandering the administration of Hap Castleton," Matt said. "If not with words, then actions. His intent is clear; the worse Hap looks; the better Wes will appear when he *'saves the hospital.'"* Matt drew the words out sarcastically.

"Wycoff and Wes have created a crisis in the minds of the board and the employees. It's nothing more than justification for a power grab."

Given Amy's feelings for Wes and her father, Matt's accusations were troubling.

* * *

That evening, Wes reflected on the events of the past seven weeks. His first priority had been to get the hospital in the black. Otherwise, the bank would pull its line of credit, and the facility would close. To eliminate losses, he could lower cost or increase revenue. Since costs are easier to manipulate in the short run than revenue, he focused on reducing costs first.

Wes began by studying the reasons for the dramatic increase in costs the industry had experienced. He visited with administrators and physicians at the University Hospital. He learned that a breakdown in the market mechanism had created disincentives for the appropriate use of healthcare resources. He also learned about *managed care*, an initiative to create incentives for physicians and administrators to control costs.

Having a better understanding of the industry, Wes then focused on specific cost irregularities at Peter Brannan Community Hospital. He found that labor and material cost per patient day were higher at Peter Brannan Community Hospital than at most of its competitors.

Satisfied with the progress that had been made, he decided that the next logical step would be to investigate the revenue side of his hospital's profit equation. Revenue is a function of volume and price. Wes decided to address the volume issue first. He had heard that St. Matt's Hospital had been successful in increasing its share of the market.

Wes called Pete Lister, the director of marketing at St. Matthews with the hope that he would be willing to share some insights on how he could increase revenue by increasing patient volume. He made an appointment for Friday.

22

The Revenue Equation

From deep inside the office, Wes listened to the gas turbine engines winding up on the Bell 230 helicopter. The pad was a short distance from the east entrance of St. Matt's Hospital. As heat from the compression ignited a mixture of fuel and air in the twin combustion chambers, the sleeping engines angrily awoke, shaking the building until the floors vibrated and the windows rattled.

Across the room, close up against the window, Pete Lister watched the Life Flight helicopter take off. Facing east, it hovered six feet above the ground while the pilot visually scanned his instruments. Then, smooth as a lazy Susan, the aircraft rotated 180 degrees west and lifted off into the icy morning sky.

"It's a marketing tool, you know," commented Pete Lister, Director of Marketing as he turned from the window. Lister retrieved a pipe from the windowsill and fished for a tobacco pouch in the side pocket of his tweed sport coat. "With two helicopters and three fixed-wing aircraft, one of which is a Cessna Jet, we drop from the sky capturing patients from all over the state—patients that might otherwise be transferred from rural areas to Timpanogos Regional Medical Center or to the Ensign Peak Regional Medical Center."

Lister opened the pouch, gently filled the pipe, and then tapped the tobacco down with his thumb. "We think our care's better, of course, and the flights are medically necessary. But they are marketing tools, still the same," he said, placing the pipe in the corner of his mouth.

A tertiary care center, St. Matt's Hospital was not a competitor with Peter Brannan Community Hospital. The marketing director was gracious enough to spend an hour to teach Wes the fundamentals of hospital marketing. Wes guessed Lister's age at forty-five. A closely cropped salt-and-pepper beard framed his square jaw. With his pipe and tweed coat, he looked more like a philosophy professor than the successful marketing director of a $250-million-a-year organization.

Lister lit his pipe. "It hasn't been long, you see, that hospitals have had to market their services. In the old days, under cost reimbursement, our physicians were able to create demand. Prospective payment put an end to that. Although I haven't studied your hospital's statistics, there are probably several reasons for the decline in patient days your hospital's experiencing.

"In Utah, DRG reimbursement reduced the average lenght-of-stay in hospitals from seven to three days. In addition, many rural and suburban hospitals experienced out-migration as patients sought hospital care in larger cities."

"Why?" Wes asked.

"Transportation systems made it easier for patients to travel greater distances to receive hospital care. Also, there's the *'bigger is better'* syndrome."

Lister returned to his desk. "The third reason is that many large hospitals have become more aggressive in marketing to rural areas. Since prospective payment systems have capped prices and reduced patient days, the only way to increase volume is by capturing patients from other facilities."

Wes was puzzled. "How do Salt Lake hospitals market to patients in Park City?" he asked.

"One way is by selling managed care programs to employers in your community that mandate the use of Salt Lake hospitals," Lister replied. "If your facility had lost the Mountainlands contract, a significant number of patients would have been channeled by employers to other inpatient facilities."

Lister's comments were consistent with Wes's observations. On his drive that morning to Salt Lake City, he saw several highway signs advertising HMOs sponsored by metropolitan hospitals. Most were directed to employers. Although HMOs were being sold on the basis of their potential for cost savings, it hadn't previously occurred to Wes that they were also an effective hospital marketing tool.

"Then what's the solution to our declining inpatient volume?" he asked.

"There are several possible solutions," Lister said. He retrieved a marketing report from his desk drawer. "The first is to recognize that, hospital patient days represent a smaller and smaller portion of total healthcare cost in the current environment. Notice the decline we've had in inpatient revenue as a percent of total revenue," he said, handing the report to Wes. "If Peter Brannan Community Hospital is to survive, it must supplement its inpatient revenue with other services."

Wes took notes attentively. "What types of services?"

"Outpatient services like laboratory and outpatient surgery, occupational medicine products, and durable medical equipment. For years physicians have been skimming—building their own outpatient surgical centers to perform high profit, low-risk procedures, while leaving the high-cost, high-risk, low profit procedures to the hospital. Hospitals have to take some of that business back."

"Give me an example," Wes said.

"LASIK surgery," Lister replied.

"Some hospitals are selling vitamins, or offering limited forms of alternative medicine," Lister continued. "That might be a new revenue source for your facility."

"What types of alternative medicine?" Wes asked.

"Meditation, Yoga, acupuncture."

"Aren't there liabilities to offering alternative therapies?"

"Yes, but in some cases, no more than for traditional treatments. You have to be selective," Lister said. "I'm not advocating crystal therapy, but some forms of alternative medicine have been shown to have therapeutic value."

Lister continued. "As insurance companies place more and more restrictions on the procedures they're willing to pay for, many hospitals have begun to market services to self-pay patients. There are shops in malls where a person can get a complete laboratory work-up without a physician's order. The stores don't diagnose, and encourage the patient to review the results with his or her physician. Some provide diagnostic services that insurance companies won't pay for. procedures that are more expensive, but less invasive than those offered by the hospital."

"Doesn't this alienate hospital medical staffs?" Wes asked.

"Yeah, but they're already alienated. Let's face it, many of your physicians are draining off your high revenue procedures." Lister looked directly at Wes. "How many of your physicians operate their own labs, x-ray machines, or outpatient surgery units?"

"I don't know."

"Check it out," Lister said. "To illustrate how innovative some providers are in marketing to the self-pay market, there are group practices that have cut out insurance companies all together. For $4,000 a year, a patient can enroll in a plan that entitles him or her to immediate telephone access to a physician, twenty-four hours a day. The patient is guaranteed a physician appointment within four hours."

"What kind of acceptance have these plans had with the public?" Wes asked.

"Within two weeks of offering the plans, many group practices have sold out. When reduced overhead due to the elimination of paperwork is factored into the formula, the physicians work less hours and make more money. Again, it is strictly for self-pay patients, there is no insurance. Hospitals could do the same thing."

"Okay," Wes said, still taking notes. "What else can I do?"

"A second approach to increasing patient volume might be to educate local employers who buy HMOs on the negative impact that sending patients to distant providers has on the local economy. As patients leave, so do their dollars. Studies show that for every dollar that leaves the community for hospital services, an additional sixty cents is lost in retail revenue.

"A third approach might be to increase inpatient volume by capturing a larger share of the local market. To do that, you might consider starting your own hospital-sponsored HMO. There are also a number of small rural hospitals in northern Utah and southern Idaho that can't offer the breadth of services Peter Brannan Community Hospital offers," Lister continued. "I suggest that you make a greater effort to capture their referrals."

✳ ✳ ✳

To learn more about pricing under prospective reimbursement,
read Supplement 4, "Pricing Products and Services."
For a detailed discussion on the design of hospital
cost accounting systems, reference the
following supplements:

Supplement 5—*Information Needs of Managers* (recommended for all students: medical, nursing, health administration and accounting)

Supplement 6—*Cost Accounting Taxonomies* (recommended for health administration and accounting students)

Supplement 7—*Designing Accounting Reports to Meet Information Needs* (recommended for health administration and accounting students)

Supplement 8—*Designing the Pricing Module* (recommended for health administration and accounting students)

Supplement 9—*Regressing RVUs to Determine Fixed and Variable Costs* (recommended for health administration and accounting students)

Supplement 10—*Direct Materials and Hospital Overhead* (recommended for health administration and accounting students)

Supplement 11—*Ratio of Costs to Charges* (recommended for health administration and accounting students)

Supplement 12—*The Use of Case-mix in Assessing Efficiency* (recommended for all students: medical, nursing, health administration and accounting)

Supplement 13—*Rolling up Standard Procedure Costs to Determine Product Costs* (recommended for health administration and accounting students)

23

The FAA Report

On Monday Dr. Irene Cowdrey was back to present the results of the compensation study. Both Wes and Natalie were pleased with a methodology that allowed them to calculate standard cost for revenue departments such as nursing. They called a meeting for department supervisors. The objective was to use these standards to develop flexible budgets.

Supervisors initially worried that the standards would be used punitively. Enthusiasm for the program increased when Wes announced that 50 percent of the anticipated saving from tighter standards would be shared with employees through an employee productivity bonus pool.

It was early afternoon when Wes returned from his meeting with his department heads. Two men were waiting outside his office. The larger one spoke first.

"I'm Officer Kuxhausen," he said, producing FBI identification. "Mr. Smith is with the Federal Aviation Administration. We'd like to visit with you privately."

Wes nodded, and they followed them into his office where he shut the door. "You're investigating Hap's accident?" Wes asked when all were seated. "Any clue about the cause?"

Kuxhausen nodded at Smith, who produced a large manila envelope.

"We have evidence that someone tampered with the plane," Smith replied. Opening the envelope, he laid two photographs on the desk taken by the FAA of the wreckage. Wes studied them, surprised that Del Cluff could have survived the accident. The impact had broken the back of the aircraft. The fire that followed reduced the fuselage to a charred skeleton.

Smith removed a pointer from his shirt pocket. "This is a picture of the right engine, taken the morning after the accident," he said, leaning over the photograph. "The cowling surrounding the engine has been removed to expose the fuel pump. The nozzle connects to the fuel hose. Note the small hole—the probable cause of the fire.

"Notice the sticky residue here," Smith continued, pointing to the fuel line. "Kuxhausen was the first to notice it—the lab tells us it's a petroleum-based electrical tape that originally covered the hole."

Wes looked up. "A fuel line repaired with electrical tape?" he asked skeptically.

"No—sabotaged. The boys at the FAA lab tell us the hole was carefully sanded with a three-sided file. Fuel pressure in a Cessna 340 comes through the line at about thirty-five pounds per square inch," Kuxhausen injected. "Whoever made the hole covered it, knowing that the aviation fuel would soften the tape, breaking the seal and allowing the fuel to escape. From the burn marks, you can see that the fuel ran back along the hose until it made contact with the hot magneto." He outlined the path with a ballpoint pen.

A menacing smile cracked Kuxhausen's face. "Clever way to bring a plane down, don't you think?"

"Not with you guys around," said Wes. "Any idea who did it?"

"Nope. That's why we're here. Are you aware of anyone who had it in for Hap Castleton?"

Wes frowned. "Everyone in the public eye makes enemies sooner or later. It's no secret the hospital's got problems—big problems. Vendors haven't been paid, employees may lose their jobs, but no particular suspect comes to mind. You're welcome to interview the employees and staff."

"We will," Kuxhausen said. Removing a business card from his wallet, he slapped it on Wes's desk. "In the meantime, if you think of anything else, give us a call."

Outside the hospital, Smith and Kuxhausen visited briefly in the parking lot before going their separate ways. "Do you think he's a suspect?" Smith asked.

Kuxhausen picked at the remnants of a steak sandwich between his teeth with a plastic toothpick. "He seemed stressed," he said. "On the other hand, what would he have to gain? Anyone who'd aspire to Hap Castleton's job isn't smart enough to sabotage an airplane."

* * *

Following Kuxhausen's visit, stories about Hap's death swept through the hospital like wildfire. Motives rumored behind the murder ranged from a crime syndicate interested in the hospital's undeveloped property to efforts of the hospital board to cover up illegal contracts they had taken to provide services at inflated prices to the hospital. One story even postulated an affair between Del Cluff and the wife of a jealous physician. Wes had trouble visualizing Del Cluff in the role of paramour, but as with all rumors, logic was irrelevant.

Wes had no idea why anyone would harm either Hap or Cluff. He was aware of a growing hostility within the community in general—and the hospital in particular—toward the financial problems plaguing the facility. The hospital had $90,000 in payables to local vendors who would not be paid in the event of a bankruptcy.

Loss of employment by several hundred employees was a similar concern. Tempers flared as employees, physicians, and board members deflected blame for what all feared was an impending financial disaster.

Though Wes didn't fear for his personal safety, he had come to the conclusion that a hospital failure would have a severe negative effect on his career. He wasn't responsible for the bad decisions that had brought the hospital to the brink of ruin, but in the community's eyes, he would share the blame—as the facility's last hospital administrator.

The advisability of circulating his resume with former associates from Portland, Maine crossed his mind. Late that afternoon, he drove to the Castleton residence to visit with Amy and Helen Castleton, where he discussed with Helen Castleton the possibility of Hap's murder. Helen had no idea of who would want to harm her husband but reinforced Amy's early observation that Hap had seemed different in the weeks before the accident.

24

An Audit of the Pharmacy

With the exception of the running shoes and trophy rainbow trout, the administrator's office looked much the way it had when Hap died. Wes didn't care for the décor. It was overdone and out of date. If the hospital survived and Wes was offered the permanent position of administrator, the velvet drapes and French Provincial furniture would go. For the present, however, there was little reason to change the décor.

Still, it would be nice to have a desk that worked, Wes thought as he struggled once more to open the top drawer, jammed for the second time in as many days. Grasping the handle, he jiggled it firmly to no avail and then hit it forcefully with the palm of his hand. Still, it didn't budge. Something was caught in the runner.

Pushing back the heavy executive chair, he retrieved a screwdriver from the bottom drawer, then climbed under the desk. From his position lying on his back, it took a moment for his eyes to adjust to the dark. The runners were covered by a 2' x 3' baseboard, securely attached to the side panels by four screws. Interestingly, an amateur carpenter had sawed an opening about the size of a legal envelope in the center. It was covered with a small door with two hinges and a small latch. *A hiding place?* Curious, Wes released the latch. A yellow envelope fell out, hitting him on the chin. Retrieving it, he crawled out from under the desk.

Sitting on the couch next to the door, he examined the penciled label on the envelope. *"Raymer Investigation."* It looked like Hap's handwriting. Inside were several slips of paper. The first was a three by five card with the name of Randall Wynn Simmons penned on it. Beneath, also in Hap's handwriting, was the inscription, "12 Percodan prescriptions, January through March 1994."

There was a 1997 invoice from the hospital to the Lycaon Home Health Agency for pharmaceuticals—sixteen cases of Sudafed. The order included four other items, all of which Wes recognized as over-the-counter drugs containing metamphetamines. A notation indicated that Raymer had paid for these items personally.

The last items in the envelope were two receipts from the hospital, both dated February 27, 1993. The first was for a topical antibiotic for $7. The second receipt was for a prescription for a drug called Ziac for $12.52. A canceled check to the pharmacy from the account of Hap Castleton for $19.52 was stapled to the back of the second receipt. Wes studied the documents for a few minutes and then picked up his phone and called medical records.

"Hi, Shannon, Wes here. Have we ever had a physician on the staff by the name of Randall Simmons? ... Never heard of him, huh? How about a patient? The full name is Randall Wynn Simmons . . . Yeah . . . check the files and give me a call.

Thanks." Wes hung up and returned his attention to the documents. In a few minutes the phone rang.

"Hi, Shannon. No one by that name ever admitted here? At least as far as the records go back, huh? And how long is that. . . Okay, thanks anyway."

There was a knock at the door and Natalie Simpson entered. "Come in," Wes said, "I was just going to call you." Natalie crossed the room and sat down. "Ever heard of the Lycaon Home Health Agency?" Wes asked.

Natalie shrugged. "I've sent them invoices," she replied. "We serve as the pharmacy for five nursing homes and three home health agencies—they're one of them. They have a post office box in Salt Lake City."

"Why do we sell them pharmaceuticals?"

"Hap authorized it four years ago. It increases our purchasing volume—we share the volume discounts."

"Who owns Lycaon?" Wes asked.

"Don't know," Natalie replied. "We just invoice them for the drugs they order, they pay their bills. We have an open purchase order from them in the file someplace."

"Why don't you pull it," Wes suggested. "I would like to see who signed it. I'd also like you to do some research on this home health agency to determine who owns them. Call the Department of Business Regulation," Wes said as an afterthought. "And while you're playing the role of detective, see if you can find out anything about a fellow by the name of Randall Wynn Simmons. He may have filled an outpatient prescription at the hospital sometime in 1994. Check these prescription numbers." Wes handed Natalie the card.

Natalie's blue eyes reflected her curiosity. "What's this all about?"

"I'm not sure, but it may have some bearing on Hap's death. See what you can find out, but keep it low key, okay?" Wes cautioned.

* * *

That afternoon, Natalie pulled the open purchase order from Lycaon Home Care. A Nancy Baum had signed it. She listed herself as the purchasing agent. The name didn't ring a bell, and she couldn't find her in the Park City or Salt Lake City phone books. She called the administrative offices of the Social Security Administration and found Lycaon wasn't Medicare certified. *Strange,* she thought, *Medicare is the largest payer of home healthcare costs in the state of Utah. How do they stay in business?*

With a visit the following day to the Department of Business Regulation, she obtained a copy of Lycaon's business license and articles of incorporation. To her surprise, the owners were listed as Ryan Raymer and Hank Ulman, both employees of the hospital. Late that afternoon, she reported back to Wes.

"As far as I can determine from talking to the offices of Medicare, Medicaid, Blue Cross, and several other large insurance carriers," Natalie said, "Lycaon has never billed a third-party payer for a visit. Yet they've run a good volume of drugs through the pharmacy over the past two years."

"Were we paid?"

"To the penny."

"Why would Raymer and Ulman own a home health agency?" Wes asked. "It's outside their expertise."

"Beats me! Neither has said anything to me about it." Natalie said.

"What about Randall Simmons?" Wes asked.

"Almost forgot," Natalie replied. "That's an interesting story in itself. I couldn't find his name in the phone book. I began to wonder if he was still alive, so I checked out the Social Security Death Index on the Internet. He died in Fillmore, Utah, in 1997. I called Millard County and got a copy of his death certificate. He passed away in a nursing home."

"I checked the phone book for the nursing home, no listing. I called the Utah Nursing Home Association and found the place burned down in '97. I was able to place a call to the former administrator. He retired and lives in Greeley, Colorado, with his daughter. He recalled Randall Simmons; said he was a patient there for four years prior to his death. He told me Simmons was a retired physician from Panguitch, Utah. Practiced from 1949 to about 1989.

"Decided to call the Bureau of Narcotics," Natalie continued. "The numbers you gave me were for prescriptions signed by Dr. Simmons in 1996—class three narcotics for a patient named Darin Erickson. No one knows who Erickson is, but they were filled at a pharmacy in Salt Lake City. Simmons' license was lifted two months later as a result of these prescriptions."

"Why?" Wes asked.

Natalie smiled cynically. "Dr. Simmons had Alzheimer's—he didn't have his mental faculties after 1994. "I wondered if Erickson was still alive, so I ran his name through the Social Security Death Index. I found a fellow with that name who died in 1966. I checked with the Drivers License Division and found that someone using his name and social security number had obtained a driver's license in 1989. Apparently, this person obtained a copy of his birth certificate from the data on his tombstone and used it for identification."

Wes was silent while he digested the information. "A physician with Alzheimer's, who writes narcotics prescriptions, for a dead man with a renewed driver's license. What do you make of it?"

"I think someone's forging prescriptions and filling them using fake ID," Natalie replied.

Wes nodded. "Good work, Natalie, keep snooping. Let me know what you find."

25

Facility Problems

Wes Douglas laid his glasses on the blueprint, then rubbed his tired eyes. He was perplexed. For the past two hours, he and his chief engineer, John Conforti, had met with Brett Patterson, Park City's Fire Chief, to determine if there was a way to bring the facility in conformance with the State Fire Code.

Wednesday, Wes received a six-page letter from Patterson's boss, the state fire marshal, detailing the building's violations. The letter threatened to close the facility unless a remedy was agreed upon. Wes immediately called Patterson to set up a meeting.

Patterson, who had done his best to cooperate, shook his head apologetically. "My own kids were born here; we come here for healthcare. We don't want to see the hospital shut down, but it's got to meet code, Wes."

Many violations had been resolved, but two remained. Wes replaced his glasses and studied the blueprint. "This main section of the building dates back to 1935," he said, tapping the document with his knuckles. "What I don't understand is why the issue's coming to a head now."

"The State Fire Code was amended in 1995," Patterson replied. "Back then, we put the hospital on notice then that the facility would have to be remodeled or closed. The board promised they'd build a new facility. With that understanding, we gave them a variance. All that changed in September when the board announced the cancellation of the project." Patterson arched his eyebrows and shrugged. "No replacement—no variance."

Wes took a deep breath, then released it slowly. He understood Patterson's argument; he just didn't have much money. "Okay," he said with a tone of finality. "I'll agree to replacing the sprinkler system. Hate to do it as the whole building will be torn down in a couple of years anyway, but you leave me no choice." Wes turned to Conforti. "How much will that cost us?"

"Fifty thousand bucks."

Wes swore softly. "What's left?" he said returning his attention to the blueprint.

"The newborn nursery."

"I can't close the newborn nursery," Wes said. "We can't survive if we get out of the baby business. Besides, Castleton just spent $30,000 recruiting and outfitting a new obstetrician."

"If you keep it, you have to get a code-approved egress," said Conforti. "The current hallway's too narrow. It's three feet wide; the code calls for ten. It met code when the wing was built but doesn't now."

"I have an idea," said Patterson. He pointed to an area near the Nursery. "You could create a new hall by removing the west and south walls of the pharmacy storeroom. That would give you a twelve-foot hallway emptying directly into the lobby—just thirteen feet from the main entrance."

Wes nodded as he studied the blueprint. "Might work," he said. He turned to

First floor, Administrative Wing, Peter Brannan Hospital

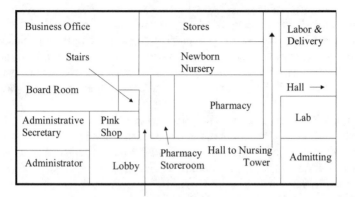

Nonconforming hall to Nursery

Conforti. "Why didn't you think of that?"

Conforti shrugged. "I don't know, but I like it. I'd rather lose a storeroom than a Nursery."

"There's one problem," Conforti continued. "Ryan Raymer's pretty possessive of the area. Two months ago, the director of volunteers tried to get it for the Pink Shop. Raymer lost his cool. Never seen anyone react that way; you'd have thought we were asking for the keys to the narcotics vault. Ask him again, and you'll probably get the same reaction."

"Then we won't ask him," Wes countered. "He's gone for the weekend, and the fire marshal will be here Monday. Let's get a crew in this afternoon. I'll deal with Raymer later."

✳ ✳ ✳

Friday afternoon, Natalie reported back to Wes on the continuing investigation of Ryan Raymer. "He becomes more interesting by the day," said Natalie. "By policy, the pharmacy must deposit all funds received on a nightly basis. Raymer has always resisted—complaining he was too busy. I'm on the board of the hospital credit union; Raymer's a member. In the past five years, he's financed some expensive things: a boat, a cabin, and a Lexus automobile. Usually, he pays the loans off early, making sometimes two or three extra payments a week. The dates always correlate with the dates on which he makes the pharmacy's deposit."

"What do you make of that?" asked Wes.

"I was puzzled by the pharmacy receipts you gave me from Hap's envelope. I wondered why they were with the other documents. The prescriptions were for medications Hap was known to be taking. There was nothing unusual about them."

"So?"

"So we pulled the cash register tape Raymer delivers with the pharmacy deposits. In theory, it is a copy of the receipts from the pharmacy sales for the day."

"Why do you say 'in theory?'" asked Wes.

"Because the dollar amounts for the transaction numbers found on Hap's receipt for that same date are different. My theory is that after the pharmacy closed and the other employees went home, Raymer would re-ring the tape with fictitious transactions, under-ringing the transactions by as much as $200 per day. He would then use that money to pay down his credit union loans. The cashier there said he always pays in cash."

"You think Raymer was embezzling from hospital?"

"Sure do. There's more. I got his Social Security number from his personnel file and used it to obtain a copy of his birth certificate. What was unusual was his mother's maiden name—*Wycoff*. That's not a common name, so I checked his pedigree with the Family History Library in Salt Lake City. His mom was the sister of your finance committee chairman, Edward F. Wycoff."

Wes raised his eyebrows. "Raymer is Wycoff's nephew? He said. "I didn't know that."

"Neither does anyone else. It's a well-kept secret."

"Why?"

"It would be interesting to find out," replied Natalie.

✳ ✳ ✳

Saturday afternoon, the carpenters removed the pharmacy storeroom walls without incident, creating a hallway between the nursery and Pink Shop. The only surprise the construction crew had was a heavy bookshelf with a built-in cabinet attached to the east wall.

"Funny, it's not shown on the blueprints; must've been added later," said the carpenter. "Shall we tear it out?"

The supervisor studied it carefully, then shook his head. "It's not a bad-looking piece of furniture," he said. "Leave it. That new night security guard Wes hired after the burglary has been griping that he doesn't have a place for his stuff. We'll move a small desk there and it can serve as his workstation. Make sure to drill it, screw it to the wall securely. There'll be considerable traffic through this area. We don't want someone with a service cart knocking the darn thing over."

✳ ✳ ✳

"What's up with him?" Paula Grable, pharmaceutical technician, asked as she opened the cash register. It was Monday morning, and as the pharmacy was about to open, Ryan Raymer had blown through the door, screaming something about the remodeling project.

"Guess they hadn't told him. He takes a personal interest in any changes to the pharmacy," she said as she opened the retail window. "Frankly, I like the change. We never used the storeroom anyway. Now the nursery has a legitimate exit if there's a fire."

"Where'd he go?" asked the other pharmacist.

"He left as quickly as he came. Started off for administration," she said with a funny look in her eye. "Swearing a blue streak, he was. Then strange . . . he stopped, about halfway down the hall . . . stood there a moment . . . white as a ghost. Looked absolutely frightened to death. Then he turned and, without saying a word, headed for the parking lot."

26

Raymer's Reversal

"Why didn't you warn me?" Raymer screamed, his rage choking him. Raymer had just burst into Ulman's office. His brother-in-law had never seen him angrier.

"Warn you 'bout what?" asked Ulman as he took his feet off his desk.

"Warn me they were going to knock the walls of the pharmacy storeroom out."

"Didn't know they did," Ulman replied, surprised as Raymer. "Why would they do that?"

"Made the thing into a hallway," Raymer replied. "Connects the newborn nursery to the lobby."

"I never saw a work order," Ulman said defensively. "It wasn't on the schedule board when I left Friday." His eyes widened as he thought about the hidden staircase, "Did they find the door to the lab?"

"I don't know—no, don't think so. The bookshelf is still there . . . but they bolted it to the wall. Worse still, they've put a desk with a phone and our security guard in front of it—now it's his workstation!"

A tense silence enveloped the room. "What are you going to do 'bout the delivery?" Ulman asked. "You promised to ship Thursday. You can't renege again. Carnavali's capable of murder."

A nauseating wave of fear washed over Raymer—for a moment he couldn't breathe. "I don't know," he gasped. As his eyes darted about the room, he wiped the beads of perspiration forming on his upper lip. "Our options are limited. We've got $55,000 worth of Sudafed down there. We can't get it out without tipping everyone off, and even if we had the money to replace it, it would take me a couple of months to do it without raising the suspicions of my drug reps. You don't order $55,000 of amphetamines without someone asking questions."

"We've got other problems here at home," Ulman volunteered as Raymer evaluated his options.

"Like what?"

"An investigation Wes has started on the home health agency."

"What are you talking about?" Raymer asked. The tension in his abdomen tightened.

"I was installing a new phone line for a computer. In the business office, you know, on Friday. Heard Natalie Simpson talking with Kayla Elmore," Ulman continued.

"Who's Kayla Elmore?"

"Accounts Receivables Clerk. Anyway, Simpson's askin' her to pull all of the home health agency purchase orders to the pharmacy. She's calling the State Division of Business Regulation in to do an audit of the agency's prescriptions."

"Why would he do that?" asked Raymer.

"Maybe they found Cluff's work papers. Maybe they were in Hap's desk. They sure as the devil weren't in Cluff's. I searched the place for thirty minutes the night I broke into the business office." Ulman shook his head. "You've got a problem, buddy."

Raymer's face hardened. "No, we've got a problem. If I go down, you go down."

27

Paradigm Software

Tuesday, Wes scheduled a meeting with David Brannan to discuss the foundation's pledge on the new facility. From reading minutes of the board of trustees, Wes learned that the Mike and Sara Brannan Foundation had committed an endowment of one million dollars for the new building. Originally, it was to be paid in four installments. The first installment was made in April of 1999, according to schedule. In June, David Brannan reported that the foundation was having financial problems, and put the board on notice that additional payments might not be forthcoming. Wes wondered why.

David Brannan arrived dutifully at two o'clock. It was apparent to Wes that he was embarrassed by the family's default. As David took a chair in Wes's office, Birdie popped her head in to remind the administrator that he was two hours behind on his afternoon appointments. The waiting room was filled with hospital creditors, physicians, patients, and unhappy employees, all demanding immediate solutions to their problems.

Wes didn't waste time on small talk. "I met with the fire marshal," he said soberly. "The building doesn't meet code. We are making some changes, but in the long term, remodeling will cost more than replacement. Unless we can demonstrate progress on a new facility, they plan on shutting us down."

"With the hospital's current financial situation," Wes continued, "and without the foundation's endowment, we stand little chance of obtaining additional financing. What are the odds that the foundation will be able to help us with the remaining $750,000 on the pledge?"

"I wouldn't hold my breath," David said. "No doubt you have been apprised of the family's financial difficulties."

Wes nodded.

"There's less than a 50 percent probability the foundation can meet its commitment," David continued. "The foundation's assets consist of 10,000 shares of Brannan Inc. Brannan Inc. is a holding company," he continued. "At its peak, it owned two coal mines, a major interest in Whittingham's bank, Park City's only newspaper, and Paradigm Systems, a software development house. All that's left is Paradigm. It's not yet profitable."

"But it does have value?" Wes asked.

David nodded. "It could. I have a potential buyer. He won't commit, however, until the company demonstrates that it can turn a profit."

As a C.P.A. with Lytle, Moorehouse, and Butler, Wes had consulted with several high-tech firms in Maine and was familiar with the industry. Many fortunes were being earned in software development. Folding his hands he leaned forward. "Tell me more," he said.

"The company was formed in 1994 by a group of engineers and software programmers in Seattle, Washington. On their first contract they teamed with Tandem Computer and an electrical engineering firm to develop and install a hardware and software system for the Boeing Corporation.

"Boeing was concerned about the security of its aircraft plant in Renton. There was a lot of union unrest—concern about industrial espionage. Boeing contracted with Paradigm for a computerized security and environmental control system. The system was to provide security, access control, monitoring, and fire protection for their entire facility.

"Employees would be allowed to access only those areas for which they were authorized. A Tandem computer would control access through the central station. One of the requirements was that it have the ability to read and process 15,000 employee access control cards during the ten-minute period employees report to work each morning.

"It was an expensive project," David continued. "The hardware included a central command post, employee identification card readers, television cameras, monitors, and smoke and fire detectors—all in addition to the software code.

"Halfway through the project, Paradigm ran out of money. They had underbid the contract. Father bought the company, thinking he could save it with an infusion of a million dollars. He was wrong; the software had a major design flaw. By the time the contract was finished, the overrun exceeded $4 million. Unwilling to lose his initial investment, Father came up with more money. The funds came from other companies owned by Brannan Industries. In retrospect, he wouldn't have bought Paradigm if he had known how much money it would take to finish the contract. He bled his other companies to get the cash."

"What's the status of the contract now?" Wes asked

"The project is finished, and there are new potential customers. Paradigm is currently negotiating with a large hospital chain to design and install a similar security system for its hospitals. This system would also include the monitoring equipment in the ICUs and nursery."

"What else is needed?" Wes asked.

"Eight hundred thousand dollars for development work. I have a venture capitalist who will fund us, but he is unwilling to put the money in until we can demonstrate our ability to control cost. If I can get the $800,000, we can modify the software and get the contract."

"Okay, so you have a computerized environmental control and security system."

"Right."

"And the software works."

"More or less. There are bugs, but I think they're minor. The system's running in Texas and Washington," David explained.

"And you have customers, with money, willing to buy and modify the system, and a venture capitalist who will fund it," Wes asked.

"Right, and an investor that will buy the company if it turns a profit."

"What else do you need?" Wes asked.

"More sophisticated control systems—specifically job order costing."

"If I could help you put an acceptable system in place, how long would it take for you to finish the contract?" Wes asked.

"About three months," David replied.

"At that time, you think you could sell the company for enough money to cover the foundation's commitment to the hospital?"

"Yes," David affirmed.

"I've developed costing systems for defense contractors," Wes said. "I don't have much time, but we can't survive without the prospect of a new hospital. I'll give you forty hours of free consulting time. Let's see if we can get Paradigm Medical Systems in the black."

David's eyes lit up as he considered the possibility of a sale. "That would be great. Wes, I need one additional favor," he said.

"Shoot."

"We are working on interfacing our computer with a telemetry unit that can broadcast a video signal at least seven miles to a central station. We need a place to test the telemetry component of the system in a reinforced concrete building. We'd like a room in the hospital."

"How large of a room do you need?"

"My engineers tell me we need a room with about four hundred square feet. There has to be at least one floor above the test room, and it needs to be within two hundred feet of other telemetry units like fetal heart monitors. We need to test for interference."

"How long do you need the room?"

"About a week."

"I'll give you the boardroom," Wes said. "Coordinate with Mary Anne."

✷ ✷ ✷

"Ryan? . . . Ryan Raymer, isn't it?" A large man wearing a convention name tag stuck out his hand. Ryan Raymer's hand remained by his side. With more important things on his mind, he was in no mood for petty conversation, especially from someone he didn't know.

"Do I know you?" Raymer asked. His lips puckered with annoyance.

"Peter Applebee. Don't you remember? The Elk's Home? Claremont, California? My wife and I are in Park City for a convention."

Raymer's eyes hardened. "Remember the school," he snorted. "Don't remember you." With that, he broke off and continued down Main Street. He didn't look back.

"My!" the conventioneer's wife asked "Who was that?"

"He was raised with me in the Elk's home—a real loner," her husband replied. "No one knew much about him. He started exhibiting bizarre behavior in the sixth grade. Became obsessed with poisons and explosives, as I recall—started experimenting. He was finally sent to a lockdown institution when the headmaster's car blew up. We never heard what happened to him after that. The conventioneer shook his head. "He was a strange kid."

"Well!" his wife exclaimed, "it doesn't seem like he's changed much!"

28

First Management Reports

Monday morning, Natalie met with Wes to review the first reports of the new cost accounting system. From the beginning, Wes's objective was to empower the department heads by giving them the information they needed to make decisions. He believed that Hap had often made decisions that should have been made on a department level.

The meeting was held in the boardroom so that all of the reports could be spread out for examination. Natalie laid the reports on the table, then stepped to the whiteboard. "When we first met with the department heads last September," she said, "they told us they needed information for . . ."

Natalie wrote on the board:

Information is needed for:

- *Pricing*
- *Cost control*
- *Strategic planning*
- *Measurement of the comparative efficiency of our hospital with other facilities*

"I think the system we have implemented will meet the criteria. For pricing," Natalie continued, "we can now produce reports showing our actual direct cost and our fully loaded (or absorption) cost by product and by product line. We can provide detail all the way down to the procedure level. For costing, we can define the product as . . ."

Natalie wrote on the board:

Product Definitions

- *A patient day*
- *An admission*
- *An employer*
- *A capitation month*
- *A DRG*

Natalie continued. "We can produce flexible budgets, showing fixed and variable costs at different levels of volume for each product definition. We have already begun a comparison of costs, as calculated by the new costing system with the reimbursement we receive under billed charges, negotiated capitation rates, and DRG payment."

"We can tell how much we make or lose by patient day, admission, employer etc. under each of those reimbursement systems?" Wes asked.

"That's right." Her mouth pulled into a frown. "Unfortunately, we're finding that revenue isn't even close to cost in some cases."

"I suspected as much," Wes interjected.

"Well, the reports confirm it," Natalie said. "For cost control, we've adopted a standard costing system that will allow us to compare actual cost to standard cost, computing the appropriate price and volume variance by product, product line, and department." She wrote on the board:

A variance is the difference between standard cost and actual cost. The new costing system will allow us to calculate price and volume variances by:

- *Product*
- *Product line*
- *Department*

"Lets look at the reports," she said, "and I'll show you how they work." The first report shows us profitability by DRG."

Peter Brannan Community Hospital
DRG Based Analysis

1	2	3	4	5	6	7	8
DRG	# of Cases	Average Lenght-of-stay/Case	Average Charge/Case	Average Contractual Adjustment Per Case	Average Net Revenue Per Case	Average Cost Per Case Per Standard Costing System	Average Profit/(Loss)
21	12	3.10	$ 8,450	$ 2,340	$ 6,110	$ 6,570	$ (460)
44	36	1.50	3,561	288	3,273	1,280	1,993
48	14	6.70	12,780	4,508	8,272	8,108	164
67	65	4.30	5,699	3,402	2,297	4,100	(1,803)
83	59	2.40	2,398	780	1,618	3,280	(1,662)
121	101	2.60	9,931	3,943	5,988	7,241	(1,253)
Avg		3.43	$ 7,137	$ 2,544	$ 4,593	$ 5,097	$(504)

Definition of Column Headings:

Column 1: The diagnostic related group (DRG).
Column 2: The number of cases in each group seen by the hospital for the period.
Column 3: The average length patients in this DRG category stayed in the hospital.
Column 4: The average amount that the patients in this DRG category would have paid if all patients were paying billed charges.
Column 5: The difference between billed charges and what the hospital was reimbursed, on average, for patients classified in this DRG for this period.
Column 6: The average actual reimbursement received by the hospital for all patients in this DRG category (regardless of their insurer, or the reimbursement system used by their insurer). This is calculated by taking actual reimbursement received and dividing by the number of patients.
Column 7: The average cost to the hospital per case using the standard costing system developed by the Peter Brannan Community Hospital.
Column 8: The average actual profit or loss on all patients seen in this DRG category (the difference between

Column 6 and Column 7).

"We make the most money—$1,993 per case—on DRG 44. We lose the most money—$1,803—on DRG 67. The average loss per case for the six DRGs shown here is $504."

"The next report," Natalie continued, "is an analysis by insurance company for DRG 125—Circulatory Disorders. We'll use this report as we negotiate with our third-party payers. Notice that 50.58 percent of our contractual adjustments come from Medicare Part A. Total cost for Medicare Part A patients for this period was $201,462. Reimbursement was only $75,777. Our write-offs totaled $125,685."

Peter Brannan Community Hospital
Payer Based Analysis
DRG 125—Circulatory Disorders

1	2	3	4	5	6	7	8
Payer	Avg Lenght-of-stay	Total Charges	Net Revenue	Adjustment from Revenue to Charges	Percent of Total Charges	Percent of Net Revenue	Average Contractual Adjustment %
Blue Cross Federal	2.0	$ 45,882	$ 42,212	$ 3,671	4.8%	7.6%	8%
Blue Cross Other	2.4	46,162	44,777	1,385	4.8%	8.1%	3%
Medicaid	2.1	75,561	40,281	35,279	7.9%	7.3%	47%
Medicare A	5.8	277,239	75,777	201,462	29.2%	13.7%	73%
Medicare B	1.3	107,329	50,230	57,099	11.3%	9.1%	53%
Ajax	2.3	226,673	190,406	36,268	23.9%	34.6%	16%
Misc. Payers	1.6	169,650	106,520	63,130	17.8%	19.3%	37%
Totals	1.6	$948,496	$550,203	$398,294	100%	100%	42%

Definition of Column Headings:

Column 1: Insurance company paying for patient's healthcare in the hospital.

Column 2: The average length a patient insured by this insurance company stayed in the hospital for DRG 125 during the period.

Column 3: The total amount the insurance companies would have paid for all patients, if they had paid billed charges.

Column 4: The actual total amount the insurance company paid for all PBCH patients covered by their plan classified in DRG 125 for the period.

Column 5: The difference between Column 3 and Column 4.

Column 6: The percent of total billed charges patients in DRG 125 insured by this insurance company would have generated.

Column 7: The percent of net revenue received paid by this insurance company for patients in DRG 125.

Column 8: The average contractual adjustment as a percent of Total Charges.

Wes studied the report for a few minutes. "The report gives a lot of information on why we're losing money," he said. "Notice that on the average we only collect 42% of billed charges. Our largest contractual adjustments are for government programs such as Medicare and Medicaid."

"Here is a similar report by attending physician for every doctor who treated DRG 125," Natalie said. "Each physician has a slightly different practice pattern. Some physicians make the hospital money, some don't. Notice that for physician 0031, we lose about $2,958 every time he treats a patient with a DRG 125 diagnosis."

Peter Brannan Community Hospital
Physician Based Analysis
DRG 125

1	2	3	4	5	6	7	8
Attending Physician	Total Cases	Average Lenght-of-stay/Case	Average Charge Per Case	Average Contractual Adjustment Per Case	Average Net Revenue Per Case	Average Cost Per Case	Average Profit or Loss Per Case
0031	20	2	$11,173	$ 5,280	$ 5,893	$ 8,851	$ (2,958)
9226	15	3	8,904	3,172	5,732	7,124	(1,392)
0906	8	3	9,294	4,093	5,201	7,349	(2,148)
1127	8	2	6,212	2,766	3,446	4,068	(622)
9735	8	6	13,222	8,371	4,851	9,911	(5,060)
0881	6	2	8,678	2,731	5,947	7,449	(1,502)
3235	6	1	6,427	1,193	5,235	4,430	805
4962	5	2	9,015	3,440	5,574	8,048	(2,474)
0483	5	1	9,513	4,729	4,784	7,644	(2,860)
0348	5	1	6,692	1,858	4,834	4,396	439
1231	4	1	5,366	1,539	3,827	3,112	715
1242	3	1	7,947	2,659	5,288	5,192	96
0321	2	4	10,678	6,470	4,208	9,354	(5,145)
6803	1	6	13,773	413	13,360	10,483	2,876
1638	1	6	16,896	2,703	14,193	11,932	2,261
3537	1	4	10,970	1,755	9,215	10,513	(1,299)
2462	1	4	12,010	961	11,049	7,623	3,426
0988	1	1	7,425	3,713	3,713	5,652	(1,939)
1232	1	12	17,195	12,992	4,203	12,212	(8,009)
Avg	101	2.60	$ 9,391	$ 3,943	$ 5,448	$ 7,241	$ (1,794)

Definition of Column Headings:

Column 1: Code number for the attending physician.

Column 2: Total number of DRG 125 patients or cases seen by attending physician.

Column 3: Average lenght-of-stay for attending physician's patients classified in DRG 125 category for the period.

Column 4: The average amount a patient would have paid for DRG if patients had paid billed charges.

Column 5: The difference between billed charges and what the average patient paid during this period.

Column 6: The average revenue the hospital actually received for all patients attended by this physician in DRG 125.

Column 7: The actual cost of treating these patients, using the standard costing system developed for the hospital.

Column 8: The average profit or loss per case for patients of this attending physician for DRG 125 for this period.

"We can use this to profile physicians. We can compare not only the resources they use to treat individual diseases, but their outcomes to determine the best treatment profiles. A physician's treatment profile can be created using a multiple regression model similar to what Dr. Cowdrey used in determining market weightings for job characteristics in the determination of salaries. As you recall, the model is

$$Y = a + b_1X_1 + b_2X_2 + \ldots b_nX_n$$

"Y indicates the percent of positive medical outcomes, the X_n's are the resources used (diagnostic tests, prescription drugs, nursing procedures, etc.), and the b_n's are the quantity, level or combination of resources used. On a preliminary basis, we have applied this model to the medical staff for seven diagnoses to determine if we have treatment outliers—physicians whose practice patterns are significantly different from those of their peers in the kinds and quantities of diagnostic tests and treatment procedures ordered. If you plot the treatment profiles on a bell curve, most fall in the center; but there is one significant exception," Natalie noted, "Dr. Matt Brannan."

"A different treatment profile isn't always bad, is it? Wes asked. "Practice patterns vary across the country. Physicians are trained at different medical schools that teach different protocols. Besides, isn't the practice of medicine continually changing?"

"That's true," replied Natalie. "That's why we regress against outcomes. If the outcomes are better, then other medical staff members can learn from the improved treatment profile. In this case, they are not. Dr. Brannan has significantly higher negative outcomes as measured by operating room complications, infection rates, and percentages of patients not having a successful recovery. The data don't tell us he's a bad physician, but it raises some flags. As soon as we verify the data, I recommend you share it with the credentialing committee."

"Not a bad idea," replied Wes.

* * *

Thursday afternoon, Natalie took the data to the University Medical Center where it was reviewed and confirmed. Friday morning, Wes met with Dr. Emil Flagg, chairman of the Credentialing Committee, to discuss his concerns. "The quality of Dr. Brannan's care has been a concern since he joined the medical staff," Emil acknowledged soberly as he reviewed the reports. "I'm not surprised at the data. He has had more than his share of complications."

"After reviewing his training, I'm no longer convinced that he's qualified for family practice. As I look at his file, certainly he applied for and received privileges in obstetrics and surgery that he isn't qualified for.. "Dr. Brannan completed an internship, but never had a residency. He's not board certified in family practice, obstetrics or surgery."

"How did that happen?"

"A rural hospital with a poor history of peer review, a father of the applying physician who has funded its deficits for the past twenty years. It was politics," replied Emil. "Hap should have been more aggressive when Brannan applied for membership on the medical staff, but I think he had his hands full with problems created by managed care, and didn't want to risk his relationship with the Brannans."

"Who grants medical staff privileges?" asked Wes. "The administrator, the medical staff, or the board?"

"The medical staff, through the Credentials Committee makes recommendations. The final power lies with the board, however. The administrator is their agent."

"After he joined the staff, Brannan ran into complications with several patients. The nursing staff is on record of having complained about him on at least two occasions. Where was the medical staff when all of this was happening?" Wes asked.

"Brannan's partner visited with Hap off the record, but was unwilling to criticize him openly as he had to practice with him. The physicians in the clinic across town also expressed concern, but felt since Brannan was a new competitor they would be accused of 'sour grapes.' Historically, physicians have been reticent to criticize their peers. It's a brotherhood, there is a tendency to stick together."

"Hap was burned several years ago," Emil continued, "when he took disciplinary action against a radiologist. Everyone on the medical staff had complained privately about him. When the administrator took formal action, however, it became '*them against us*.' The staff rallied behind the radiologist."

Wes removed his glasses and absently stared out the window as he collected his thoughts. "Okay, so what do we do now?" he asked.

"Dr. Brannan will be meeting before the Mortality and Morbidity Committee next week. It will be his second time before that group in less than a year." Flagg was silent as he counted his power chips. The Brannans were no longer funding the hospital. Several members of the medical staff owed him favors . . . it was time to call in the political IOUs he held.

"With a new administrator," he said almost as though he were talking to himself, "and a renewed resolve on the part of the board to fix the hospital, this very well may be the time for me to push for a resolution." He turned to Wes. "It's not that I've been a laggard in the past, it's just that the problem has political ramifications, and the environment in the past wasn't favorable."

"If there's a fight among the medical staff, it won't be pretty," Emil continued. "And you'll be right in the middle, taking sword blows from all sides." He looked Wes straight in the eyes. "When there are problems, the hospital administrator's makes a pretty good fall guy. The community can't fire the board, and they don't want to fire the medical staff, and so . . ."

"I get your point," Wes said. "No need to finish the sentence."

"Let's be candid, Wes, when the board went after you they wanted a hired gun. To do the things that need to be done to save this place you'll make lots of enemies.

The board would be crazy to stand someone as unpopular as you're going to be in certain circles. You're too new to have many allies. Once the dirty work's done, you're expendable.

Wes was quiet while he absorbed the message. "Wish I'd have known this when I was offered the job," Wes said. "I guess I could have figured it out if I'd thought it out."

"Welcome to Politics 101," Emil said. "So, what do you want to do?"

"Let's do the right thing," Wes said.

* * *

Monday afternoon, Dr. Emil Flagg reported back to Wes. "The committee restricted Dr. Brannan's obstetric and surgical privileges," he said, "but rejected the proposal to suspend him from the medical staff. Their recommendation is that he go back and get a residency."

"What was his response?" asked Wes.

"He'll live with the restricted privileges; he has no choice, although he's angry about it. At this point, he has no interest in returning to school."

"The problems we are having with Dr. Brannan are raising the issue of quality in general," Wes said. "I'd like to meet with someone who is doing research in the area to see if there is anything we can do to improve the overall quality of our product. Total Quality Management (TQM) and Continuous Quality Improvement (CQI) are big issues in manufacturing, and I think they deserve evaluation in healthcare as well."

"There are continual studies being done on those topics at the University of Utah Medical School," Emil said. "If you want, I'll see if I can get someone down here to talk to us."

"Let's do it!" replied Wes.

29

Improving Physician Decisions

Dr. Tom Woolsey's eyes sparkled with approval. "Your interest in quality is timely," he said. He and Dr. Crystal Hammond were in the office of Wes Douglas at the request of Dr. Emil Flagg. Both Woolsey and Hammond were professors. Woolsey taught biostatistics and epidemiology in the department of preventive medicine at the University of Utah Medical School. Hammond was a professor of business administration at Weber State University. At Wes's invitation, Dr. Emil Flagg and Dr. Ashton Amos were also present.

"I met Hammond at a symposium on marketing sponsored by the Healthcare Marketing Association," Woolsey said. "Much of what she had to say related to my interest in total quality management. We have subsequently coauthored several articles on that topic together." Woolsey turned to Hammond. "Why don't you begin by reviewing your research?"

Crystal Hammond, a stocky woman in her mid-thirties, cleared her throat. "There are four stages in the competitive evolution of markets," she said. "The first stage can be summarized by the phrase *"If you build it, they will come."*[3] In this stage, demand exceeds supply, and the power is in the hands of the provider with the greatest number of assets."

"In the healthcare industry, this occurred in the 1950s," Woolsey added. "The country was concerned about a shortage of hospital beds. The federal government intervened with funds through the Hill Burton program for the construction of new hospitals."

"Our 1956 wing was built with Hill Burton money," Dr. Amos volunteered.

Hammond nodded, and then continued. "In the second stage, demand catches and then exceeds supply. Firms begin to compete in the marketplace. This is the stage of selling and competition. In healthcare, this occurred in the early 1970s. Hospital beds alone no longer guaranteed success. Hospitals began marketing their services, although cost reimbursement softened the impact of oversupply.

The third evolutionary stage is a period of restructuring. The focus is on eliminating excess capacity. We have seen this in retailing, banking, and manufacturing . . ."

And the healthcare industry," Woolsey injected. "Look at what's happened over the past decade as hospital corporations have purchased and downsized competing facilities. The focus has been on the elimination of duplicate facilities."

---

[3] Berkowitz, Eric N., Ph.D. and Robert T. Kauer, Ph.D., "The Strategic Life Cycle," *The Journal of Strategic Performance Measurement,* August/September 1998, Volume 2, Number 4.

Hammond nodded. "The final stage is customer value," she said. "Finally, the seller focuses on quality. That's where the health industry is today."

"Several factors are motivating a new emphasis on quality," added Woolsey. These include:

- Employees who are concerned about having their physicians and hospitals mandated by their employers.

- Increased access to health information through the Internet.

- An appreciation for the success manufacturing has had in improving products through total quality management (TQM) and continuous quality improvement (CQI)."

"What are the major medical centers doing to improve the decisions of their medical staff?" Wes asked.

"Some are studying how physicians arrive at a diagnosis," Woolsey responded.

"I participated in a study that borrowed from research done by business schools in human information processing," Hammond said. "This study focused on:

- Physician memory
- Cue weighting
- Problem definition
- Hypothesis formulation
- Information search

"What is *cue weighting*?" asked Dr. Flagg.

"A cue is a piece of information that assists the physician in determining the true diagnosis," Hammond answered. "A cue could be a medical symptom, a vital sign, the result of a laboratory test, etc. A physician typically evaluates many cues in determining the diagnosis. *Cue weighting* is concerned with the importance the physician attaches to each cue. One can actually demonstrate the physician's decision model through the equation:

$$Y = a + b_1X_1 + b_2X_2 + \ldots b_3X_3$$

Where the Xs are the cues and the bs or betas are the weight or importance the physician attaches to each individual cue. Show them your model," Woolsey said to Hammond.

"It's not actually *my* model," Hammond said. "It's an adaptation of the Brunswick Lens Model. Accounting researchers use it to study how the users of accounting information make decisions." She walked to the chalkboard and drew the following diagram:

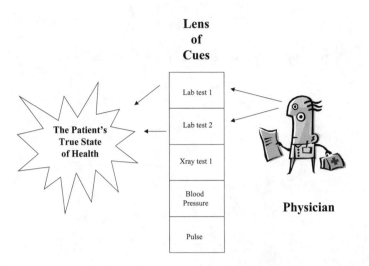

"The physician, on the right side, cannot see the patient's true state of health. To determine that, the physician must therefore view it through a lens of cues. These are signals that help determine a diagnosis. These include the results of laboratory and x-ray tests, vital signs such as blood pressure, the patient's pulse, etc."

"The actual cues used by the physician and the weights placed on each of those cues constitute the decision model. As Woolsey said, this decision model can be mathematically formulated. To show how that's done, let me expand the diagram." Hammond then drew the following:

Regression Formulation of the Lens Model

Cues

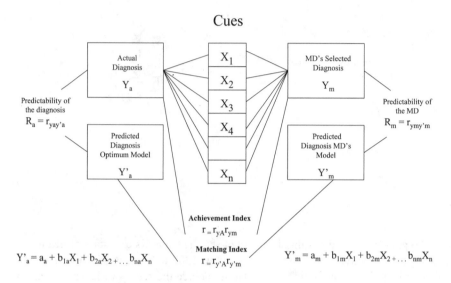

"In this model, the cues are designated by the notation X_1, X_2 . . . X_n. Y is the diagnosis, and the bs or betas are the weights or importance the physician places on each individual cue. As Woolsey said, the decision model can be written mathematically as:

$$Y = a + b_1X_1 + b_2X_2 + \ldots b_nX_n$$

"In the regression formulation of the lens model, we are concerned with four decision models. $Y_m = a_m + b_{1m}X_1 + b_{2m}X_2 + \ldots b_{nm}X_n$ in the upper right box is the model the physician *actually* uses. I don't have space to write the entire equation, so I only wrote Y_m in the box. Again, Y_m is the diagnosis the physician finally settles on, the $X_1 \ldots X_n$ are the signals or cues he relies on, and the bs or betas are the weights or importance the physician places on each of the cues."

"What do the subscripts mean?" asked Amos.

"The *"m"* means that it is the MD's model, and the numbers are just ways of differentiating the betas and cues," Hammond replied. "Medical schools across the country have interviewed physicians to determine what their model is. They have done this by asking the physicians what cues they look at in determining a diagnosis and how they weigh these cues. The physicians' *stated* decision model, in the lower right hand box, is written as

$$Y'_m = a_m + b_{1m}X_1 + b_{2m}X_2 + \ldots b_{nm}X_n$$

140

Flagg was confused. "What's the difference," he asked?

"People don't always do what they say—their actual behavior doesn't always follow their model."

"Why?" Flagg asked.

"Because they're human. They get tired, they get hurried, they don't feel well, or maybe they're in a bad mood because they had an argument with their husband or wife. The notation

$$R_m = r_{ymy'm}$$

signifies the degree of correlation between Y_m and Y'_m. It tells us how consistent the physician is in using his or her own model—how predictable his or her decision-making behavior is."

"I wouldn't want to go to a physician who wasn't consistent," Wes replied.

"Neither would I," said Hammond. "That's one reason for collecting the data to perform the correlation."

"Okay, so what do the boxes on the right side of the cues indicate?" asked Flagg.

"Y_a represents the actual state of health or diagnosis of the patient. We use the subscript *"a"* to designate the *actual* diagnosis. If we knew everything about how the body works (which we never will), the model for determining the correct diagnosis would be

$$Y_a = a_a + b_{1a}X_1 + b_{2a}X_2 + \ldots b_{na}X_n$$

"Since medical science doesn't know everything there is to know, this is differentiated from Y'_a (pronounced *Y prime a*) which is the diagnosis the physician would arrive at, if all current medical knowledge were used. This diagnosis would be determined through the decision model

$$Y'_a = a_a + b_{1a}X_1 + b_{2a}X_2 + \ldots b_{na}X_n$$

"Can you ever determine that Y'_a was not Y_a?" asked Wes.

"We try to do that through autopsies. Also, as medical science learns more, we are sometimes able to retrospectively make that determination from the medical records of past patients."

Flagg's face lit with recognition. He was getting the hang of the notation. "Then

$$R_a = r_{yay'a}$$

tells us how good the very best decision model currently available to medical science is in determining the correct diagnosis?"

"It signifies that correlation!" said Hammond. "Now, if we want to determine how close the physician's decision model is to the optimum decision model (given the current state of medical knowledge), we calculate the correlation between Y'_a and Y'_m. That is designated on the chart by the notation

$$r = r_{y'_a r Y'_m}$$

"We call that the matching index. It tells us if the physician is following the best practices in determining the patient's diagnosis."

The correlation obviously isn't very high for Dr. Matt Brannan, thought Flagg. *It would be nice to have this information on all of our medical staff so we could determine who needs further education.* Dr. Flagg returned to the original list of factors.

- Memory
- Cue weighting
- Problem definition
- Hypothesis formulation
- Information search

Flagg smiled with satisfaction. "I think I understand cue weighting," he said. "And *problem definition* is self-explanatory; it is the identification of the patient's complaint. Now, tell me about *hypothesis formulation.*

"Hypothesis formulation takes place when the physician identifies possible causes of the patient's problem—the list of possible diagnoses," replied Hammond.

"I saw an interesting study on that very topic in the *Journal of the American Medical Association (JAMA),*" said Amos. "It reported that physicians who identify the right diagnosis in their list of possible diagnoses almost always select the correct final diagnosis. Physicians who select the wrong diagnosis do so because they don't initially generate an adequate number of hypotheses."

"They stop too early in identifying the potential cause of the patient's problem?" Flagg asked.

"That's right," Amos replied. "They don't spend enough time formulating alternative hypotheses."

Flagg's face reflected his interest in the subject. He leaned forward. "That's not the end of the process, however," he said. "Having identified the correct diagnosis, a doctor must then select the optimum treatment."

"That's right, and you could also use a regression model to signify the proper combinations of medical inputs:

$$Y_o = a_o + b_{1o}X_1 + b_{2o}X_2 + \ldots b_{no}X_n$$

"Y_o would signify the outcome, given the current state of medical knowledge. The Xs would signify medical inputs (prescription drugs, surgery, hospitalization, physical therapy, radiation therapy, etc.), and the betas would signify the appropriate levels or amounts of those resources."

"This leads us to the topic of outcomes management," Hammond said. As this is Woolsey's expertise, I'll have him explain it to you."

Woolsey stepped to the board and took the chalk from Hammond. "Using medical outcomes to assess provider decision models has been around for a long time," Woolsey said. "This approach was proposed in 1913 by a Harvard surgeon by the name of Emery Codman. He called it the *end results idea*. It consisted of tracking surgical patients for a year to see how their treatment turned out. The objective was to determine the most likely cause of success or failure. Codman planned to accumulate the information into a database that could be used to improve treatment profiles. Unfortunately, his proposal to the American Medical Association was essentially ignored—it received only $500 in funding. More importantly to Codman, other physicians stopped sending patients to him, his practice suffered, and, as a consequence, he abandoned the idea.[4]

"In 1919, the concept was resurrected by the American College of Surgeons that performed a study of 692 hospitals with 100 beds or more. The study showed that only 89 met the minimum standards. The response of the Board of Regents to the report was swift and uncompromising. They collected all the copies, carried them to the basement of the hotel, and burned them."

"The regents were obviously men of action," Flagg said with a sarcastic laugh.

"Despite its rocky beginning," Woolsey continued, "outcomes management is receiving attention again due to pressures of employers and consumers who would like to be able to judge the quality of the healthcare services they are receiving. One approach is to build clinical pathways, physician guidelines, and treatment protocols. Though this approach has its critics, it also has its supporters.

"Research conducted by a number of medical schools has shown that there is a large geographical variation in treatment patterns among physicians. Patients like to think their physician's approach is based upon what research has shown works best, but unfortunately that isn't true. Physicians don't always follow the best practices. The result is that resources are wasted, and, in some situations, patients actually die. A 1992 Harvard study estimates that as many as 180,000 patients die each year from medical mistakes.[5] A 1997 Rand Corporation study of autopsies shows a 35 to 40 percent error rate in diagnoses."[6]

"Why don't physicians follow the best practices?" Wes asked.

"There are two schools of thought on that one," Woolsey said. He wrote the following on the chalkboard:

- *Physicians don't know what the best approaches are.*

- *Physicians get bogedg down in dealing with the tremendous volume of information needed to make decisions.*

[4] Many of the concepts in this section is drawn from an excellent article by Joey Flower entitled "Measuring Health," which appeared in the *Journal of Strategic Performance Measurement*, August/September 1998, Volume 2, Number 4.

[5] Allen, Jane E. "Doctors, Insurers Meet to Highlight Ways to Reduce Medical Errors," Associated Press, October 14, 1996

[6] "U.S. Health Care Can Kill, Study Says," *San Francisco Chronicle*, October 21, 1997

"Let's address the first possibility," Woolsey said as he retrieved a professional journal from his briefcase. "Part of the problem is that we don't know what the best practices are."

"That's hard to believe," said Wes.

"Let me read from an article in the August/September *Journal of Strategic Performance Measurement,*" replied Woolsey. "Most practices in clinical medicine have never been tested in double-blind peer-reviewed scientific studies, or even through retrospective statistical analysis. When practice techniques have been firmly established or debunked in such studies, the knowledge often does not seem to affect clinical practice. Many physicians fail to hear of the new knowledge; others routinely ignore it, preferring to continue to practice the way they were taught in medical school."[7]

"The first problem can be solved through research and education," Woolsey continued. "The second problem is caused by limitations in human memory."

Hammond spoke. "Studies on human information processing indicate that we have two types of memory. Long-term memory is almost unlimited in its capacity, while short-term memory is limited to six or seven chunks of data. Unless a physician follows a decision tree when making decisions that involve multiple variables, it is easy to get confused and wrongly weight the cues."

"But we have the technology to supplement short-term memory," said Wes. "PC computers can store, organize, and retrieve an almost unlimited amount of information."

"That's right," Hammond replied. "And a number of teaching hospitals have developed decision-tree software programs for use by physicians in the diagnosis process. Unfortunately, not all physicians have embraced that technology. Many still rely on memory."

"I think we have pretty well covered the theory," Flagg said. "Now let's be more specific. What can the medical director of a small hospital like ours do to improve the quality of its physician decisions?"

"There are several things you can do," replied Woolsey. "Your quality control committees can start performing outcome audits.

You can encourage members of the medical staff to adopt practice protocols that have been shown to have the best outcomes. These are essentially pathway guidelines, as opposed to boundary guidelines that define medical practices beyond which physicians incur penalties. You can also encourage physicians to use existing computer technology to store, organize, and retrieve these protocols. The use of computers to retrieve and execute decision trees can reduce errors resulting from omissions of memory."

"What can hospital administration do?" asked Wes.

"You have installed a cost accounting system that will identify the medical resources used to treat patients. You might consider including outcomes data in your database."

---

[7] Flower, Joe. "Measuring Health," *The Journal of Strategic Performance Measurement,* August/September 1998, Volume 2, Number 4.

Wes nodded as he took notes.

"You can also adopt many recent innovations of manufacturers in the areas of continuous quality improvement (CQI) and total quality management (TQM)," offered Hammond.

"Your initial focus," she continued, "should be on, improving customer satisfaction, market share, and profitability. It should also focus on eliminating waste and rework and on improving productivity The most important part of this program will be the management of the core processes within the hospital—processes that have been shown through double-blind randomized clinical trials to improve outcomes."

"To really work," Flagg said, "the system will have to be clinically meaningful. That means we will have to gather and report clinical data."

"That's correct," said Woolsey. "One community hospital I'm consulting with has begun by identifying four high-volume critical medical conditions for outcomes assessment." He walked to the board and wrote the following:

- *Pediatric asthma*
- *Pregnancy*
- *Cardiovascular disease*
- *Acute myocardial infarction*

"Could we hire you to help us do the same?" Flagg asked.

"Dr. Hammond and I would be happy to help you in any way we can," Woolsey replied.

"Where will we get the money?" Wes asked.

"That's your assignment," said Flagg.

30

The Competition

With the successful completion of the first module of a cost accounting system, Wes turned his attention to the competition. One of the obvious reasons for the decline in patient volume was Snowline Medical Center, ten miles to the south. From visiting with Logan Harker of the Utah Healthcare Association, he learned Consolidated Healthcare of Arizona, a for-profit hospital corporation formed in 1985, had built the facility.

Wes was told that the company was well capitalized and that most of its facilities were new. The company boasted saving from centralizing the purchasing, housekeeping, financial, and dietary functions. Its charges were slightly higher than many not-for-profit hospitals in the state—not including Brannan Memorial Hospital, which had raised prices in its struggle to remain solvent.

Logan reported that the company was vertically integrated, owning hospitals, nursing homes, and a health insurance company that served as the nucleus for its managed-care program. The corporation had recently started an aggressive program of physician practice acquisition in an attempt to control physician referrals.

Although the corporation had been criticized for its aggressive marketing practices, Logan was impressed by its efficiency and financial strength. She suggested that Wes meet Jon Einarson, the local hospital administrator. At Wes's request, she called Einarson and set up the appointment.

✻ ✻ ✻

"Today's hospital employees are too expensive," Jon Einarson snarled. At age thirty-five, he stood six foot three and tipped the scales at a muscular two-hundred-twenty pounds. His closely cropped beard accentuated the rawboned features he inherited from his Icelandic ancestors, and his sea green eyes could pierce an opponent like a Viking pikestaff.

For the past two hours Einarson had given Wes a tour of his building, highlighting efficiencies in design that allowed the hospital to reduce staffing by 20 percent. Now both dined in the private dining room adjacent to Einarson's office. Einarson reached for his steak knife. "A good administrator knows how to slash labor costs," he said cutting the rim of gristle and fat from his thick steak. "That's why we axe old facilities. We design our buildings to save labor. In five years we can pay for a new building in payroll savings alone.

"Prior to entering the market," he continued, "I approached your board with a purchase offer. Your finance committee chairman, Edward Wycoff, killed it." Einarson took his first bite and nodded approvingly as he savored the flavor. "It was a mistake," Einarson continued. "Park City would have been a better location for us, but your board resisted our for-profit ownership. In the long run, the decision will hurt us both."

"Why?" asked Wes.

"Because there isn't a big enough population to support two new hospitals. That's why I was pleased when I heard you wanted to meet with me. Hopefully, you've come to the same conclusion," said Einarson.

"The board will never support a consolidation," said Wes. "The community tradition is too strong."

"The tradition is wrong," Einarson retorted angrily. "Hospitals are too expensive to plop in every community along the Wasatch Front. What your board is doing is a disservice to the community. If you want to do the right thing for Park City and yourself, you'll work with us. We can make it worth your time."

"What do you have in mind?"

Einarson swallowed, then wiped his face with his napkin. He leaned forward conspiratorially, dropping his voice to a whisper. "You don't have to take explicit steps to sabotage the operations. Your hospital's a sick patient, Wes. Remove the life-support systems, and it will die on its own."

"What specifically are you suggesting?" asked Wes.

"We've heard about your efforts with budgeting, cost accounting, etc. Don't waste your efforts. Let nature take its course."

"And if I do as you suggest?" Wes asked.

"When the hospital closes, there will be a position for you with Consolidated Health Systems, at a generous salary. We'll give you a two-year contract at $150,000 a year. You won't have to do anything; use the time to rest, or find a new job."

"Three hundred thousand dollars to close the hospital," Wes mused. "What you're talking about sounds like a bribe."

"Don't get caught up in semantics, Wes. When the place falls apart, you'll need a new job. Wycoff's not going to take responsibility for the stupid things the board's done. When he gets done with you, you won't be able to get a job in Park City waiting tables."

Wes was surprised at the boldness of Einarson's offer. Jon Einarson hadn't risen to the top of his profession by being timid. Wes believed that what Einarson was proposing was a conflict of interest. Wes paused in mock seriousness as though considering the offer. "You don't mind if I discuss your generous offer with my board?" he asked.

Einarson saw through the sarcasm and was offended. "Don't be stupid, Wes. We must be discreet. I'm doing my best to save your hide, and you're insulting me."

Wes Douglas folded his napkin and placed it on the table. "Thanks," he said as he rose to leave, "but I'm not interested."

"You'll be sorry," Einarson said.

"Perhaps."

"Quote me, and I'll deny it," Einarson said as Wes left the room. Wes closed the door behind him.

* * *

Thane Ford swore—not a soft, mealy-mouth cuss like his grandmother used when she burned the rolls or dropped a stitch in her knitting, but a blaspheming imprecation that fermented angrily in his guts and exploded with the violence of an Irish pipe bomb. Slightly ashamed, he glanced over his shoulder to see if anyone was listening. That wasn't probable since the newspaper office was empty. It was 4:00 a.m. He was about to miss the deadline for the Wednesday edition of the *Park City Herald*. The press was broken—*again*.

He grabbed a rag from the table and wiped his hands. It wouldn't be easy to fix this time. Manufactured in 1952, parts were hard to get, and money was tight. Subscriptions were down. It wasn't enough that national papers like *USA Today* targeted rural markets. Even the statewide newspapers like the *Salt Lake Tribune* had online editions that stole readers from the smaller biweekly rural newspapers.

At 6:00 a.m., he'd call Edward Wycoff, his silent partner. Wycoff would write a check to fix the press—but not to replace it. Ford doubted he would ever get that commitment. There would be a price, of course—not just the verbal abuse. Ford could take that, but Wycoff would require more. Ford would agree. If it were a question of ethics or of feeding his family, he would choose the latter. There weren't other options at his age.

31

Power of the Press

Wes was elated. All morning he'd worried about the interview, and with good cause. Since assuming the post of administrator, the local newspaper had been unrelenting in its criticism of Peter Brannan Community Hospital. In a small town, hospitals operate in a fishbowl. Whenever news was slow—which was quite often in rural Utah—someone at the *Park City Herald* started poking the hospital's closets for a skeleton.

As Wes watched the front steps of the hospital, Thane Ford unlocked the door to his car. He turned and waved at Wes with a smile before entering and driving off. *Won that one!* Wes thought.

Thayne had disarmed Wes from the start. Contacting Wes's former employer in Maine, Ford had checked his consulting references. "Their enthusiasm was overwhelming," Ford reported sheepishly. "They liked your style. Said you were good at identifying operational problems, and better still at fixing 'em. 'A real smooth cookie,' one reported."

"Sorry I've been so tough on you in my editorials," Thayne continued. "It's to everyone's best interest for you to succeed—at least if we want to have a hospital."

"Volume is down," Wes volunteered, "and the negative press hasn't helped."

Thayne's eyes narrowed with regret as he stared at the floor. "In the news media, we get carried away sometimes, maybe to the detriment of our communities." His face brightened. "Tell you what we'll do," he said. "Whenever a new president is elected, the press typically gives him a sixty-day honeymoon—a period during which they lay off the negative press. Maybe we ought to do the same for you."

"That'd be great. I'll tell you whatever you want to know—so you don't think I'm hiding things from you. Give us sixty days to get our act together. If we haven't fixed things by then, you're free to go after us."

"You're a tough negotiator," Ford said. Both laughed.

"Okay. Now tell me what's going on," Thayne began. "Is it safe to be admitted to Peter Brannan Community Hospital?"

"Certainly," replied Wes. "We have our problems, like everyone else, but the overall quality is as good as any rural hospital in the state."

"What kind of problems?" Thayne queried.

"We have a physician we are disciplining. The board has temporarily suspended his privileges."

"Anyone I know?" Thayne pressed.

Can't give the name," Wes replied, "but we're working the problem."

"Any trouble getting the medical staff to support you?" Thayne asked while taking notes. "I've heard some doctors are reticent to criticize peers."

"You said this was off the record?" Wes verified, nodding at the notebook.

"It's just for the files," Thayne replied.

"There was resistance from some members of the medical staff," Wes said, "but Dr. Emil Flagg, chair of the Credentialing Committee, handled the situation."

"I hear there's quite a bit of conflict on the board."

"I don't think we want to address that publicly," Wes said warily.

"Remember the deal," Thayne said. "It's just between us."

Wes nodded, and for the next thirty minutes he answered Ford's questions about the operation of the hospital as truthfully as he could. Topics discussed included board politics, and the problem small hospitals have competing with the resources and specialized staff of larger facilities. *He probably didn't learn anything he didn't already know,* Wes thought as he concluded the interview. *Most of these problems will be fixed in sixty days; they'll be of little interest to the newspaper then.*

"I've enjoyed the interview," Thayne said as he closed his notebook. "It's given me new hope for the future of the hospital. Let's keep in touch; I need to know what's going on, but I'll support you—at least through the honeymoon period."

Standing on the steps of the hospital, Wes was elated to have found a friend and supporter. He was about to receive the shock of his life.

* * *

In the security of his office, Thayne Ford reviewed his notes. The most interesting part of the interview was the malpractice scoop—the issue that had caused the medical staff to suspend *"Dr. X."* The young administrator wouldn't tell him who that was, but at about that point in the conversation, Wes had been called into the hall to talk to a fire inspector.

Thayne took the opportunity to look at the notes of the Credential Committee meeting that Wes had referred to. As Thayne had suspected, the name of the physician had been scratched out. The patient's admission number had not been erased, however, and Ford wrote it in his notebook.

He picked up his phone and punched in the phone number of Patricia Fielding—'Trish.' Trish was a medical records librarian in the hospital and one of Thayne's sources. He had met her in a bar on her first night in town from Brooklyn. Crazy hair, but good figure.

"Heyyy, Trish! Guess who?"

The voice at the other end of the line bubbled with excitement.

"Thayne? . . . Howya doin'?"

"Doin' good. Got a favor though. Got a hospital admission number . . . wanna know who the patient is. Yeah, I can wait." He doodled on the notepad while she checked the files.

"Britanny Anderson? Seen in the emergency room, huh? What was the problem? Hmm . . . the doctor had missed the diagnosis? Almost resulted in her death? Yeah, that's bad. Family plan to sue? Well, maybe they'll change their mind," he said, scribbling in a pad. "Who's the Doc? *Ah,* Dr. Brannan . . . the *Little Prince . . . "*

Thayne Ford held his notepad at arm's length as though admiring a beautiful work of art. A big Cheshire grin spread across his face. "I owe you one, baby."

32

Anniversary Dinner

Dr. Emil Flagg smiled with satisfaction as he gazed at his wife and the children that gathered around the table. It was not often that the whole family was together. Tonight they were celebrating his sixtieth birthday, and all were here for dinner at the Yarrow Inn. It was to be a surprise party, and Emil had played the part well. Having been married to Edith for thirty-five years, however, there were few surprises. Edith never forgot an important occasion, and he knew she wouldn't forget this one. As he gazed at her, she radiated back the love that had kept the family together through the good times and the bad.

Emil was not the easiest man to live with. His impatient and explosive personality often put him in conflict with his sons, who had inherited their mother's aversion to conflict. Edith was the magnet that kept them together; and tonight the boys were here for her, as much as for him.

Robert, the oldest son, was an electrical engineer from Seattle and had flown in that evening with his wife and three sons. *A handsome family*, Emil thought. Seated across the table were Tommy and his fiancée, Megan. Age twenty-eight, Tommy had just been accepted to George Washington Medical School. It was high time that he take a bride, and Megan couldn't have been a better match if Emil had picked her out himself.

Tom and Megan had met last summer in Hawaii. Emil was presenting a paper at the annual meeting of the American College of Pathologists and had taken the family with him. Tom and Megan met at the hotel pool.

Megan's father was the president-elect of the college. Already, he had approached Emil about the chairmanship of an important committee. An honor Emil hadn't sought, it would mark an important milestone in his career. Technically proficient, Emil was never politically wired. Some of his colleagues said it was his abrasive personality. Emil believed it was his unflinching honesty.

A good pathologist doesn't use euphemisms. He wouldn't call a tumor a cyst to make someone feel better, yet that's what often happened in the world of hospital politics—incompetence was couched in softer terms in the reports of peer review and credentialing committees. Emil silently scowled. *Incompetence is incompetence—spare the euphemism!* Earlier that week, he had been in an explosive altercation with the other members of the Credential Committee over the surgical privileges of Dr. Matt Brannan.

Brannan was not board certified, and twice within the past year his lack of training got him into trouble. True, he was the youngest member of a family that had faithfully supported the hospital for two generations, often reimbursing year-end deficits from family coffers. Money, however, shouldn't be the driving force in decisions about the practice of medicine. If Dr. Brannan wasn't competent, he shouldn't have certain privileges—maybe he shouldn't even be a member of the medical staff! On this final point, other members of the staff differed. Emil prevailed. He smiled with satisfaction as he remembered the meeting.

Across the room, a tall gentleman with gray hair entered the restaurant with his wife. It was Paul Jameson, an attorney and a first cousin to Edith. *He's not here for the party,* Emil thought. Emil and Paul had not spoken for years. The distinguished couple was shown across the dining room by the maitre d' and seated at an adjacent table.

"How are you this evening, Paul?" Emil said, startling the old buzzard. Emil even stood and shook his hand. "I'd like you to meet Tommy's fiancée, Megan."

Paul hadn't seen Emil and his family when he had entered the restaurant and was surprised at Emil's cordial response. "How do you do, Megan?" he sputtered.

"I've been wanting to come by and settle that easement problem," Emil continued, before Paul could catch his balance. Paul and Edith owned adjacent cabin sites in the High Uintas north of Kamas, Utah. They had inherited the property from a common grandfather. Edith got the west section, near the highway—Paul got the east. Both pieces of property had water and timber. Paul's had a better view of the valley but lacked one important thing—access to the road.

If their grandfather had been an attorney like Paul, he would have divided the property north and south, or at least would have provided a legal access to the road. He wasn't, though; he was just a poor sheepherder who wanted to do something special for his grandchildren.

Shortly after the inheritance, Paul approached Emil about the problem. All he wanted was a ten-foot easement through Edith's property. Emil was still smarting, however, about a lawsuit Paul's client had filed against the hospital. Emil wasn't affected personally, but the case was without merit, and Emil told him so.

When Paul refused to drop the case, Emil took offense. An argument ensued in which Paul suggested the best way to reduce malpractice suits was to eliminate incompetent doctors, and Emil countered that the ethics of attorneys was one step above that of the Mafia. For ten years, they hadn't spoken, while the property sat vacant.

Paul's forehead arched suspiciously. "How much money do you want?" He asked.

Emil smiled generously as he put his arm around Paul's shoulder. "I don't want anything except to put this bitter saga to rest. Bring the papers by my office Monday. I'll sign them."

Emil's wife raised her eyebrows in pleased surprise. "That was nice of you, Dear," she said, when Emil was reseated. "I know his children have dreamed about building a cabin on the land for many years. I'm proud of you for putting an old feud behind you."

Emil shrugged good-naturedly. "If it makes you happy, it makes me happy," he said, placing his hand on hers.

"It's been a good year," he continued as he scanned the table. "Tommy's been accepted to medical school and has a lovely fiancée. Robert is doing well with Boeing, and his children are growing up to be fine boys. In addition, in November we had the largest volume in pathology ever. It's time to share our good fortune with others."

Indeed, things were getting better at the hospital. Emil had been suspicious of Wes Douglas from the start. *What did a CPA know about running a hospital?* Still— his analytical approach and never-give-up attitude were having a positive effect.

Patient volume was up and cost was down—thanks in part to a new cost accounting system Wes had installed. Best of all for Emil, the board and medical staff were—at least for the moment—not at each other's throats. There was even talk of resurrecting the building program that had been canceled shortly before Hap's death. Emil smiled with satisfaction.

A young man in a white shirt and black bow tie arrived at the table and nodded at Emil. "I'll be your waiter tonight," he said. "The house special tonight is chicken Jerusalem with artichoke hearts. It comes with a green salad with a light vinaigrette dressing."

Emil looked at his wife. "It sounds good to me, Dear," she said. "I'll take the same," he replied, without even looking at the menu.

"Maybe we should build a cabin too," Edith said, as the waiter moved down the table to take Robert's order. "We'll be having more grandchildren in coming years; it would be nice to have a family retreat."

"Even if the kids don't use it, it might make a romantic getaway for us," Emil said with a wink. Edith's brown eyes registered pleased surprise—romance was not Emil's strong suit. "As a matter of fact—" Emil's sentence was cut off by a pat on the shoulder. Looking up, he saw Thayne Ford from the newspaper.

"What a fortunate coincidence catching you both together!" Thayne said, nodding at Paul Jameson.

Emil's eyes mirrored confusion as he studied Paul, then bounced a quizzical look off Thayne.

"You two are going to be spending quite a bit of time together the next few weeks, what with depositions and all," Thayne continued.

"What are you talking about?" Emil asked.

"Haven't you heard?" Thayne chortled. "Matt Brannan is suing the hospital for public defamation of character. Paul is his attorney. As chairman of the Credentials Committee, you are listed as a defendant. It's here in tonight's paper." Ford held up the nightly edition of the *Park City Sentinel*. The headlines read: *Wes Douglas Spills All—Dr. Brannan's a Quack, Board's Incompetent.*

Flagg gasped. He grabbed the paper, spilling the ice water on his wife. She stood up, knocking her chair over, which tripped a waiter, who spilled a large Caesar salad on Paul. Flagg glared at the headlines, read the first three paragraphs of the article, then swung angrily to face Ford.

"When did Wes say this?" he snorted.

"Copyrighted article from an interview at the hospital yesterday," Thayne replied brightly. He pulled a stenographer's pad from his pocket. "Do you have a statement to make?"

"Be careful," Paul said from the adjacent table. He was wiping salad dressing from his coat with a linen napkin. "Anything you say can be used against you in the courtroom."

Emil's face flushed red. Jumping up, he grabbed Paul by the coat lapels. "I'll give you a statement—you two-faced SOB!" he shouted.

"Careful," Edith said. Emil looked at her, and then shoved the frightened attorney into the buffet table, which collapsed onto the floor, taking Paul and Emil with it.

Thayne Ford snapped a picture.

"Tomorrow's lead story," he said to himself brightly.

33

Last Official Act

Wes Douglas reached for the last pile of vendor checks Birdie Bankhead had given him before leaving for the evening. Unless a miracle occurred—which was unlikely, approving them for payment would be his last official act as administrator of Peter Brannan Community Hospital.

Downstairs in the cafeteria, the joint meeting of the medical staff and board had begun—he had been specifically asked 'not to attend.' In a few minutes, Dr. Emil Flagg would present a resolution from the medical staff to the board requesting that they release the hospital administrator. Edward Wycoff would read it, then move that the board accept the resolution. Another member of the board, probably David Brannan, would second the motion, and Wes would be history.

Wes removed his phone from the hook. A story like this hadn't hit the community since the silver mine explosion of 1910. He wasn't in the mood to talk to reporters. Picking up the pen, he started signing the vouchers and then leaned back in the large leather chair that once supported Hap Castleton. He stared at the evening edition of the *Park City Sentinel* on his desk. *Why did Thayne Ford do that?* Not only had he broken his word by immediately publishing everything, but he badly distorted what he'd been told. Wes would never call Dr. Brannan a *quack* or the board *incompetent*. The motivation had to be more than a good story.

Wes shook his head as he retrieved the pen and started signing again. He was embarrassed—embarrassed for the board that had trusted him with their hospital and embarrassed for the medical staff who, despite their imperfections, were doing their best to provide a high quality of healthcare to the residents of Park City. But most of all, he was embarrassed for the employees who deserved more than the ridicule the *Park City Sentinel* was heaping on them and their organization.

He smiled sadly. One person he would not have to be embarrassed for was Amy Castleton—she was capable of holding her own. The afternoon the paper hit the streets, she cornered him in his office. Choked with anger, she read aloud Wes's derogatory *"quotes"* about her father. Wes tried to tell her that Thayne Ford had fabricated them, but she wasn't listening.

"Father may not have been a polished CPA," she said, her eyes glistening with tears, "but he was honest . . . and he treated people with dignity." She slammed the door behind her as she left.

From the window, Wes observed her leave the hospital with Matt Brannan in his Mercedes. Wes was in love with her, but there was no way the relationship was going to work. Wes signed the last check and placed it on top of the pile. Birdie would retrieve and process the checks in the morning. There was nothing left now but to pack a few personal belongings.

He removed a pen set he had received when he left Lytle, Moorehouse and Butler and a book of poetry Kathryn had given him. From the locked bottom drawer of his desk, he retrieved the file he had accumulated on Ryan Raymer. He would mail it to the district attorney later that evening.

Downstairs the meeting was heating up. He could hear the shouting all the way up the stairwell. *It's all over but the screaming,* he thought. There was no reason to stick around; if they needed him, they could reach him at his apartment before he left town.

Heavy with fatigue, he stood and snapped shut the briefcase that held the few belongings he would take with him. Picking it up, he crossed the room, and then paused at the door. Several days earlier, he had found a picture of Amy. Hap had apparently misfiled it with an old financial report. It was taken when she was eleven years old, on a fishing trip with her father. He returned to the desk, opened the top drawer, and placed it in his side pocket without looking at it. Shutting the drawer, he crossed the office, locking the door on the way out. He would leave the keys at the switchboard.

34

Carnavali

Ryan Raymer's hands were still shaking as he unlocked the door to his Lexus at the Salt Lake Airport. He and Hank Ulman had finished a meeting with Barry Zaugg, Sid Carnavali's drug runner and sometimes-hit-man. Carnavali was ticked, and Raymer was frightened. Carnavali had paid $30,000 for drugs Raymer had still to deliver. Thanks to Wes Douglas, the lab and the raw materials were sealed away.

Zaugg had been unsympathetic to Raymer's story. As he left, he slammed a wrench through the cockpit window of the small private plane Ulman was servicing. "Worse things than this will happen if Carnavali doesn't get his shipment," he said.

Raymer slipped into his car and settled into the heavy leather seats, deep in thought. Problems were multiplying faster than he could find solutions. As he pulled out of the parking lot and onto the freeway, he realized that his life, and perhaps those of his family, were riding on his ability to solve the problem.

* * *

By morning, Raymer had a plan. He and Ulman discussed it as they ate their lunch privately in his office. "We've got three objectives," he began. "Satisfy Carnavali, retrieve the materials from the lab if possible, and get rid of the evidence uncovered by Cluff. I still think there are work papers out there, someplace. If Simpson hasn't found them, she will."

"Natalie is onto something," Ulman affirmed. "The past couple of days she's been hanging around maintenance, asking lots of questions. I think she knows about the home health agency."

Raymer nodded. "I've got a plan that will solve all three problems. Carnavali wants drugs; he doesn't care what kind. I've got fifty, ten cc bottles of morphine, another 70 bottles of Demerol in the narcotics safe that I could give him. It's two weeks' worth of hospital inventory."

"But you get audited on that stuff, don't you?" Ulman asked.

"That's where you come in," replied Raymer. "Several years ago, I moonlighted at a nursing home in Salt Lake. One night the place burned; I don't know how the fire started, but it provided the cover for me to process an order for drugs that I was able to sell on the streets.

"You want to burn the hospital down?" Ulman asked incredulously.

"Just the administrative wing. It would destroy the pharmacy, evidence of the lab, and hopefully Cluff's work papers," Raymer said.

"What about Natalie?"

Ramer shrugged. "Maybe she perishes in the fire."

Ulman was silent as he mulled the thought in his head. "No good," he said. But maybe I got a better idea. How 'bout an explosion? I've been tellin' administration for two years that the boiler's got troubles, that someone's going to get hurt or worse if they don't fix it. It's right beneath administration, and close enough to the pharmacy. It probably would take out the whole wing if I rig it right."

"Is the boiler big enough to destroy all the evidence?"

"We've got two hundred gallons of gasoline in maintenance for the backup generator. The fire marshal told us to get it away from the generator. I'll put it in the storeroom in the basement; if anyone asks, I'll tell 'em that Wes told me to do it."

Raymer reviewed the proposal in his head, then smiled and nodded in acceptance.

"When do we do it?" Ulman asked.

"Saturday morning, a little after 7:00 a.m. It's the monthly meeting of the board. With Wes gone, Simpson will be representing administration."

"What about the stuff in the lab? You gonna let it blow?"

"Friday night we get it out. We either tunnel through the wall in the basement or go down through the floor of the Pink Shop."

"The Pink Shop would be easier, it will be closed; the wall in the basement is too close to the cafeteria."

"I'll meet you tomorrow night at the Pink Shop—provided, of course, that gives you enough time to rig the boiler."

"I can do it in an hour," Ulman said. "One more question—what about your uncle, Edward Wycoff. Won't he be at the meeting?"

"He's in Denver, finalizing the details on the closure of the hospital. We're going to simplify it for him," Raymer said with a smile.

*　*　*

The mood was sober at the Castleton household. In the past four months Hap had died, a murder investigation had ensued, the hospital's financial problems were revealed, Matt Brannan's hospital privileges were suspended, and now Hap's replacement had been fired.

It was Friday evening, and Helen Castleton and Amy were finishing a quiet supper. "Your father would never have allowed things to deteriorate at the hospital like they did under Wes Douglas," Helen said, as she cleared the dishes from the table.

"Mom, to be perfectly honest, Dad *did* allow things to deteriorate," responded Amy, surprised that she was willing to criticize her own father. "He did a great job for many years, but he didn't adjust his style to accommodate the demands of managed care. The hospital's financial problems aren't all Dad's fault, but he played a role."

"At least he was never vindictive," her mother replied. "After all the Brannans have done for the hospital, to single out Matt like he did . . ."

"Whatever Wes's mistakes, he's gone," Amy said sadly. "He's closed his CPA practice and has probably left town."

"Do you think the hospital will close?" Helen asked.

"I don't know. If it does, a substantial piece of Park City's history dies with it."

"Our family has a lot invested in that hospital," Helen added.

"I know. Some of my happiest childhood memories were the Saturday mornings I spent with Dad at the hospital when he would check the mail and catch up on paperwork."

"I remember those days," Helen said. "I always thought you'd be bored to death. What was there to do while he worked?"

"Dad had one of the carpenters build a playhouse in the old safe room, below his office. They furnished it with a small table and chairs that they built in the carpenter shop."

"I didn't know there was anything in the basement but the cafeteria and boiler room," Helen replied.

"You couldn't access it from anywhere but the administrator's office. There was a small stairway behind a bookshelf in the closet. Originally, that's where they kept the payroll."

"Is it still there?"

"I don't know; I'm not even sure where to look for it. Dad's old office became a pharmacy storeroom when they remodeled the administrative wing. It would be interesting to know what happened to the small furniture, though."

"Is the storeroom still there?"

"No, that area is part of the new hall to the newborn nursery." Amy's eyes flickered with curiosity.

"That's strange," she mumbled. *"Where are the stairs?"* Amy was silent for a moment as something Wes said about Raymer started to make sense.

"What did you say, dear?" Helen Castleton asked as she finished the dishes.

"Nothing," Amy replied.

* * *

Standing in the remodeled hall outside the nursery, Amy tried to reconstruct in her mind the original administrator's office and the placement of the stairs leading to the old safe room. *Assuming that the pharmacy wall is the same, Dad's desk must have been about here,* she thought, standing in the middle of the hall. *The room was about twelve feet wide . . . that would place the closet and the stairway about where the display shelf is. The shelf isn't new; it looks like it's a remnant from the storeroom days, and it must have been used to seal the entrance.*

Moving closer she examined it. *Certainly the pharmacists must have known about the safe room. On the other hand, not many people were allowed in there; Raymer was always so possessive of the area . . .*

Her thoughts were interrupted by the muffled sound of hammering from the direction of the Pink Shop. From the space under the door, she noticed a light. Retrieving her keys, she unlocked the door to investigate.

With the exception of the toolbox on the counter, the room looked the same as when she had closed the Pink Shop earlier that evening. Crossing the room, she examined the tools, then noticed the hole in the floor, six inches or so behind the cash register. The cash drawer was empty. Quietly, she walked behind the counter and looked through the hole into the room below—*my old playhouse!*

Careful not to be seen, she looked closer. Someone was down there, assembling a cardboard box. The room was the same as she remembered but was now cluttered with tables and bottles connected with tubing that resembled a chemistry set. *Who is down there and what is he doing?*

There was a noise behind her and she turned, startled. In the doorway to the Pink Shop stood Hank Ulman in filthy coveralls. His hair was covered with chalk dust, and he was holding a crowbar. Ulman smiled, exposing his chestnut colored teeth.

"Well, it's little Amy Castleton," he chortled. "And she's come to play house."

35

The Boardroom

The fear tightened in Natalie's stomach as she studied the faces of the other members of the board. Directly across the table, David Brannan peered anxiously through a pair of broken glasses perched precariously on his nose. Ryan Raymer had been kind enough to replace them—after punching him squarely in the face. To the left was Edward Wycoff, hands securely tied behind his back. Wycoff's eyes reflected terror, stark and naked. Natalie didn't understand. *Wycoff is Raymer's uncle. . . Isn't he in on this?*

Natalie had never studied Raymer carefully before. With his coarse cranial features and darting black eyes, Raymer reminded her of a trapped animal. *So Raymer was responsible for Hap's death. I should have suspected him earlier. What does he plan to do with us?*

✱ ✱ ✱

Natalie's stares irritated Raymer. He swore under his breath and checked his watch. *"Twelve minutes. . ."* he whispered to himself *"then the fireworks start. Ulman should have been back by now; hope he knows what he's doing."* Ulman had made one last trip to the boiler room. *"Back or not, in another eight minutes I'm out of here."*

Cocking his gun, he laid it on the highly polished boardroom table. He retrieved a small bundle from his coat pocket and unfolded it, placing its contents next to his revolver—one syringe and three small vials. *Too bad Wycoff showed up. Meetings must have finished early.*

Breathing heavily, he removed a handkerchief from his shirt pocket and wiped the sweat from his face. *Strange twist of fate, really. Uncle Ed . . . the final victim of his own hatred.* Picking up one of the vials, he held it to the light. *Whole thing wouldn't have happened if Cluff hadn't stuck his nose where it shouldn't have been.* He snapped the head off the vial, nostrils flaring as the pungent odor wafted in the air. *Cluff is gone . . . in a few minutes, they'll all be gone.*

Hands trembling with anger, Raymer rotated the vial between his thumb and forefinger to dissolve any remaining crystals, and then picked up the syringe. *Coroner'll never pick this up,* he thought, *if there's anything left to autopsy.*

✱ ✱ ✱

Sergeant Pete O'Malley's frown dug deep furrows into his sunburned forehead. "Darndest thing I've ever seen," he said. He stared into the video monitor, scratching the scruff of his beard. "It don't look like no joke to me."

For the past four minutes, Sgt. O'Malley, Frank Davis, chief engineer of Paradigm Systems, and Wes Douglas had watched Ryan Raymer take over a meeting in the boardroom of Peter Brannan Community Hospital. Frank had spent the previous day installing a video security system at the hospital and had arranged a demonstration Saturday morning with O'Malley in the basement of the City Hall.

Wes was there at the request of David Brannan as Paradigm's consultant—his last assignment before leaving Park City. O'Malley picked up the dispatch radio in his office. "Unit Seven."

The scratchy response was immediate. It was officer Charlie Thurgood. "Unit Seven here."

"Charlie, I think we have a hostage situation at the hospital. I'm in the middle of a demonstration of a video security system here, and on the screen we see this guy burst into the boardroom with a gun. Sgt. Mason is off today, but Fuller's directing traffic on Main. Pick him up and then head over to investigate. I'll call the sheriff for backup. I'll see ya there."

"I'm rollin," Charlie said.

O'Malley spoke into the dispatch radio again. "A large fellow in a blue maintenance uniform may be implicated. He was in the room with the hostages but just left on an errand. See if you can intercept him before he returns."

* * *

Five minutes later the phone in the boardroom rang, just as Raymer began to fill the first syringe. Since Natalie Simpson was the only hostage who didn't have her hands tied, Raymer motioned with his gun for her to pick it up. She complied.

"Boardroom." Face expressionless, Natalie listened for what seemed like an eternity, and then held out the phone.

"It's for you," she said.

Raymer's jaw dropped. "For me? Who is it?" he whispered.

Natalie said nothing, and Raymer took the phone.

"Hullo," Raymer said, his eyes wide with curiosity.

"Ryan, this is Sergeant O'Malley." O'Malley chose his words carefully. Suspecting that Ryan Ramer was emotionally unstable, he purposefully kept his voice calm. "There are officers at each exit from the hospital, including the one leading from the boardroom to the hall. Throw your gun out and release the hostages. When the room is empty, come out slowly with your hands high above your head. We will give you further instructions at that time."

Raymer squinted at the floor with disbelief. *How did they know? Was it Ulman? That doesn't make sense. He's in as deep as I am. It must be Amy Castleton. Maybe she escaped and the police were waiting for Ulman when he went to arm the boiler.*

"Stay on the line," Raymer said. He needed time to think. *If the police nabbed Ulman before he armed the boiler, then the clock isn't ticking. There's time to negotiate. If not, I've gotta get out of here.* He lifted the receiver to his ear.

"Lemmie talk to Ulman."

"Ulman's busy."

"Then unbusy him," Raymer said, "or I start shooting people." He discharged the gun through the door. Immediately they put Ulman on the phone.

"It's me."

"Did they get you before or after the errand?" Raymer asked.

Knowing that their conversation was being monitored, Ulman was tight lipped. "After."

Raymer swore under his breath. "How did they know we were here?"

"Dunno."

"Have you told them anything?"

"Won't talk to no one but a lawyer."

"Good." Raymer paused, concerned that the conversation was being monitored. "Do you think they know . . . about the surprise?"

"I can't tell, but I want outta here!"

"That's enough," O'Malley said, taking the phone back. "The building is surrounded, Ryan. Throw your weapon out and release the hostages."

"I'm not goin' to prison," Raymer whispered to himself. "I grew up in a boy's home; I know what institutions are like."

"I have three nurses in here and four of the babies from the nursery."

"We know better," O'Malley said. "You have four hostages, all members of the board."

Raymer searched the room for a camera, but couldn't see anything. "Okay," he said. "I'll trade three of the hostages for a car. The fourth is going with me."

"Is there a bomb?" O'Malley asked.

"No."

"We know there's a bomb, Raymer. You told the hostages there would be an explosion. Where is it, and does it have a timer?"

Raymer's eyes searched the room. *How do they know? Is the place bugged?*

"I'll tell you about the bomb when I have the car," he said. "I have a cell phone."

O'Malley persisted. "When is the bomb set to go off?"

"It isn't. It's armed or disarmed by radio." Raymer lied. "There's an electronic safety device," he continued. "I have to be at least three miles from the hospital to arm it. Give me three miles and if no one is following me, I'll disarm the bomb."

The phone was silent while O'Malley conferred by radio with a SWAT team that was coming in from Salt Lake by helicopter. The estimated time of arrival was three minutes.

"You want a car, and you plan on taking a hostage with you?" O'Malley affirmed when he returned to the phone.

"Right."

"We'll get the car. Stay on the line."

* * *

Several minutes earlier, O'Malley and Wes Douglas met Officer Thurgood in the cafeteria, where Thurgood had first detained Ulman. On the way over, Wes informed Thurgood he had received a phone call from Helen Castleton earlier that morning. Amy had not returned home last night. Wes suspected that Raymer had something to do with her disappearance and worried about foul play.

There was a speakerphone in the dietitian's office; O'Malley had used it so Ulman could listen when he called Raymer. "You heard the conversation," O'Malley said to Ulman. "Raymer says there's a bomb, but no timer. Nothin's ticking; no reason to worry, right?" Ulman said nothing. O'Malley noticed that Ulman was perspiring profusely.

Ulman looked at the clock and then at the sheetrock wall that separated the cafeteria from the boiler. "I'm hot; let's go outside," he said.

"The temperature's sixty-eight," O'Malley said, pointing to the thermostat on the wall. He turned to Officer Thurgood. "I'm not hot. How about you Charlie?"

"Actually I'm kinda cold," Thurgood said with a nervous shiver.

"I've got a medical condition. It's too hot in here for me. Take me out," Ulman pleaded.

"The hospital's a good place to be if you aren't feeling well," O'Malley said. "Would you like me to call a nurse?"

"Tell us what's going on," Thurgood said, tiring of the small talk.

Ulman's voice was tight. "I'm not talkin' to anyone without a lawyer. I have a right to be taken downtown."

O'Malley raised his eyebrows. "The only lawyer in town is Phillip Thornton. He's the Little League coach. It's Saturday morning, and he doesn't like to be disturbed during practice. We'll wait here and call him at noon." O'Malley put his feet on the table and looked at his watch. "We got plenty a time."

Wes heard the whomph whomph of the helicopters as the SWAT team landed in the parking lot. Ulman looked at the clock again, the fright clearly reflected in his eyes.

"Okay, okay . . ." Ulman said. "There's no time for the attorney. The boiler on the other side of that wall is going to blow in another five minutes. It shouldn't hurt the nursing units, but it will take the whole administrative wing! You can't stop it. The room's booby-trapped from the inside. Now get me outta here!"

"O'Malley was immediately on his feet talking to the SWAT team by radio. "Get the hostages out—*NOW!*" he shouted.

Wes Douglas, pumped full of adrenaline, grabbed Ulman by the throat and threw him against the wall. "Helen Castleton called this morning; Amy went to the hospital last night, never came home. Where is she?" He screamed.

"In a room," gasped Ulman, "below the floor of Pink Shop. We dug a hole and—"

"Take him!" Wes shouted as he shoved Ulman at Thurgood. "I'll be back . . . " he started to say, but his voice was obliterated by the sound of an explosion in the boardroom.

165

36

SWAT Team

Sergeant Chapman was recruited out of high school to pitch for the Pirates. He was good—no, he was fantastic! Within seven seconds of the call from O'Malley, he threw the concussion bomb right where he wanted it—through the heavy glass of the boardroom window and onto the center of the large maple conference table. *You're out!* he thought as he dove for cover.

The detonation blinded and deafened everyone in the boardroom. It was temporary, but before the sound died, four members of the SWAT team burst through the heavy maple doors, disarming Raymer and pinning him to the floor.

Downstairs, Wes Douglas, who had been knocked to the ground, was on his feet and up the staircase to the Pink Shop. Kicking the door in, he found the hole Ulman had described, covered by a 3' x 3' square of plywood. In an instant, he climbed through it, handing Amy up to a SWAT team member who had followed him from the hall. "Hit the fire alarm!" he shouted as he emerged from the hole, hoping it would evacuate the building before the explosion.

With four minutes to go, Wes, O'Malley, and three members of the SWAT team searched both floors of the administrative wing for Saturday employees, while other officers checked to see that the ICU Nursery had been emptied. In the distance, Wes heard *"Code Red, Code Red, Code Red"* over the intercom as the switchboard activated the fire and disaster plan.

Amy and the board members were being taken a safe distance from the hospital. Raymer and Ulman were under the watch of the deputies. Running down the hall Wes thought of the nursing units housed in a separate wing to the south. Unless Ulman's bomb was a blockbuster, only the administrative wing would blow. He said a prayer for the nurses and patients.

With less than a minute to go, Wes and the three remaining officers broke through the French doors of the administrator's office, crossed the lawn, and dove into an empty irrigation canal. The explosion from the boiler room was heard all the way to Heber.

37

The Dedication

Two years later—

The local population couldn't remember a more beautiful Fall. An early chill had turned the soft Kelly green of the aspen to shades of crimson, gold, and orange. As thirty-two-year-old Parker Richards stepped from his car onto the sidewalk of the new Peter Brannan Community Hospital, it occurred to him that the festive colors were a harbinger of a new era for Park City. Only recently completed, the new hospital would be dedicated in less than two hours.

Richards was well prepared for the position for which he had been hired. After completing a degree in accounting and an MBA in healthcare administration, he served as an administrative resident at the Mountainview Hospital in Las Vegas, Nevada. His preceptor, Mark Howard, president of the American College of Healthcare Executives, was an able administrator and an effective teacher. Parker Richards's arrival in Park City was timed to coincide with the dedication of the new hospital.

The building is certainly modern, he thought. *As different from the old facility as the twentieth century would be from the twenty-first. Fewer hospital beds, more outpatient services, a helicopter pad, and telemetry that linked the ICU to the University of Utah Medical Center.* Richards had only seen pictures of the old facility. An explosion and fire had destroyed its administrative wing in 1999. No one had died, and fortunately the injuries were minor.

Crossing the lawn, he entered the modern lobby and took an elevator to administration on the third floor, where Birdie Bankhead, who had just been promoted to administrative assistant, met him. "Welcome," she said. "We're happy you could make the dedication. It's appropriate—a new hospital and our first assistant administrator. Wes is still meeting with the board. I'm sure he will be out in a few minutes."

She handed Parker a program for the dedication. "While you're waiting, you can look at this. Beautiful drawing, isn't it?" she said, pointing to the architect's rendering on the cover.

"I'm on my way downstairs to check on seating for the dedication," she continued. "If you need anything, Mary Ann will be happy to help you. You might congratulate her, she's just been promoted to administrative secretary."

Mary Ann looked up from her new desk and blushed.

"Congratulations to both of you," Parker said.

Birdie picked up a bouquet of flowers that had been delivered for the speaker's podium and hustled off to the elevator. Parker took a seat and studied the program. An introduction and welcome was to be offered by Wes Douglas, administrator. A musical number by the high school band was next on the program, followed by remarks by David Brannan, representing the Brannan family. The hospital had been made possible by a generous contribution from the Brannan Family Foundation, funded by the family's prospering software company.

As Parker finished reading the program, David's brother, Dr. Matt Brannan, entered the room accompanied by a lovely young lady. She was carrying a three-month-old baby. Parker had seen Matt on the picture of the Brannan family that hung in the new boardroom. He was told that Dr. Brannan was finishing a residency at Johns Hopkins Hospital in Maryland and would be joining the staff in another year. Parker hadn't, however, met the lady.

Mary Ann stood and greeted them at the door, hugging both of them.

"Parker, I don't think you have met Amy," she said taking the baby. "She is the daughter of our former administrator, Hap Castleton." Parker reached out and shook Amy's hand.

"And this is Hap Douglas."

Mary Ann continued, holding the baby up. "Oh yes, Amy is Wes's wife." Richards looked puzzled.

"Amy and I were childhood friends," Dr. Brannan explained. "With family and staff tied up with preparations for the dedication, she was nice enough to pick us up at the airport. My wife, Kayla, and I flew in for the dedication. Kayla is coming over with her mother."

The administrator's door opened, and David Brannan and Wes Douglas emerged. Wes and Amy embraced as Mary Ann continued to hold the baby.

"How's the residency?" Wes asked shaking hands with Matt.

"Be done in a year," he said.

Birdie returned with a cameraman from the *Deseret News*. "We need a picture for the paper," she said. While Wes Douglas, David Brannan, and Parker Richards lined up by the architect's model, Mary Ann made small talk.

"I understand you've taken up flying," Mary Ann said, addressing Matt.

"I have!" Matt replied. "It provides a good diversion from studying. As a matter of fact, I'm picking up a new plane tomorrow in Salt Lake City. Before flying back to Baltimore, I hope to take Wes in it on a fishing trip."

"Hold still," the cameraman said as he snapped the picture. He took two more.

"Where to?" Parker Richards asked when the cameraman had left.

"McCall, Idaho."

Matt took the baby from Mary Ann and held him high above his head. "It was a favorite spot of this little fellow's grandpa. Who knows," Matt continued, making a funny face at little Hap. "Maybe I can turn your workaholic dad into a first rate fisherman."

Wes smiled graciously. "It would be nice to take a break," he said, "and someday I would like to learn to fish." He shook his head as he put his arm around Amy. "But as for flying to McCall tomorrow, I think I'll just stay here and keep my feet on the ground."

With that, the group was off to the dedication.

Epilogue

It was 7:30 a.m. as the small Cessna Skyhawk 172P pulled onto the taxiway leading to Runway 16 Left. The pilot, Dr. Matt Brannan, turned COM 1 to 118.3 to check in with the tower.

"Citation jet five miles inbound. Hold for arriving aircraft," the tower instructed. Matt applied the brakes and stopped the aircraft short of the runway. To the north, the Citation jet, now at 7,000 feet, turned on its landing lights.

Matt throttled the aircraft to 1700 RPM to check the magnetos. The RPM drop didn't exceed 125 RPM—everything was in order. The Citation jet was now three miles out, its landing gear down and engines on idle. Once more, Matt reviewed his checklist: *brakes, flaps, carburetor heat.*

Matt was happy that, after considerable arm-twisting, Wes Douglas had consented to join him on the fishing trip. It would give them the opportunity to mend some fences. If Matt were going to return to the hospital after his residency, he would want a better relationship with the administrator.

Wes, through the medical staff, initiated the action that forced him to apply for a residency. Now, two years into the process, Matt saw that it was the best thing he had ever done. Even his bitterness over losing Amy was gone. The first week in Baltimore, Matt had attended church and ran into Kayla Elmore, the skinny college girl with braces, from the business office. Only Kayla was no longer in college, the braces were gone, and her mature figure was anything but skinny.

Matt had never paid her much attention at Peter Brannan Community Hospital, but she had blossomed into the prettiest girl he had ever seen. Kayla was working at Baltimore Community Hospital. They dated for a year and were married.

The Citation jet landed and turned left onto the taxiway.

"Cessna five-seven Zulu cleared for takeoff. Fly heading 320, climb to one three niner, contact departure on 124.3," was the response from the tower.

"Ready?"

Wes smiled nervously and gave Matt a "thumbs-up."

"Cessna five-seven Zulu, rolling." Matt released the brakes, pushed forward on the throttle and began his take-off roll. As the plane left the runway, both Matt and Wes thought of Hap Castleton. Three years ago, he had begun this same flight, and the tragedy that had followed had set into motion a series of events that had changed both of their lives.

History would not repeat itself. Matt and Wes would complete the trip for Hap, and the experience would be the beginning of a better relationship between two professionals who would contribute significantly to the quality of healthcare in their communities.

Wes Douglas would eventually tire of the hassles of managed care, refocusing the direction of his hospital from primary to specialty care. Capitalizing on the genetic engineering breakthroughs of the first decade of the twenty-first century, the Brannan

Genetic Endocrinology Medical Center would become regionally known for the implantation of cultured pancreatic beta cells in the treatment of insulin dependent diabetes.

In later years, Wes would serve as the president of the American Specialty Center Association and would contribute to the quality of healthcare and reduction of costs through the development of similar high-volume specialty centers throughout the country.

Dr. Matt Brannan would return from his residency. As the focus of the hospital changed, he would leave Park City for a general practice in Montrose, California. Unlike Wes Douglas, he would never gain regional attention; but would be remembered in the hearts of his patients for the quality of his care and the sincerity of his compassion.

Appendix One

Technical Supplements

In addition to the following supplementary materials, questions, problems, lecture notes, and PowerPoint slides on each of the chapters can be found on the author's web page. Go to http://www.traemus-books.com.

Instructions on receiving instructor's materials (lecture notes, PowerPoint presentations, and answers to problems) can also be found at the same address.

Supplement One

Cost Accounting in Healthcare
From the Daybook of Wes Douglas—September 27, 1999

Several years ago, I developed a habit of keeping a daybook to help me remember the technical details of important meetings. Since my appointment as interim administrator of Peter Brannan Community Hospital, I have encountered a number of new issues that I thought would be helpful to record for future reference.

Lack of Viable Cost Accounting—Effect on Operations

One issue I will have to address is the installation of a cost accounting system. The importance of this project was illustrated during my first meeting with the board of trustees this morning, the meeting at which I was hired as interim administrator.

Half way through the meeting, Wycoff was upbraiding Selman for the hospital's poor performance when Helen Ingersol, a new member of the board, interrupted. Helen owns a successful construction firm that she and her husband formed before his death.

"I'm not an accountant," she said, addressing David Brannan, "but this is the first time I've seen the hospital's financial statements, and there are a couple of questions I need answered before I decide if I'm going to stay on the board."

"Shoot," Brannan said.

"Mr. Selman, your financial report indicates that the hospital's volume is up . . . but so are its losses. Your costs haven't increased dramatically—in my business that would signal that the problem is pricing. How do your prices compare with those of your competitors?"

"We aren't sure," Selman replied. "We have a copy of the competitions' billed charges. The problem is, no one pays billed charges anymore. Increasingly, hospitals are paid under prospective payment systems, more commonly called PPS. The payment under prospective payment is either mandated by the insurance company or determined through competitive bidding. Last year we bid on a large prospective payment system contract with Mountainlands Insurance, and frankly, we're losing our shirt on it."

Prospective Payment Systems

"What's a prospective payment system?" she asked.

"A payment system where the price is set prior to rendering the service," Selman replied.

"It's essentially a fixed-price contract?"

Selman nodded. "That's right."

"How were you paid before PPS?"

"Some payers, the largest of which was Medicare, paid us under a *cost reimbursement system*. At the end of the year, their auditors would determine our actual cost per patient day. If they had paid more than costs during the year, they received a refund. If they had paid less, they sent us a check."

Ingersol's eyes flashed with recognition. "As a contractor, I understand the advantages of cost reimbursement contracts and the risks of fixed price arrangements. The key to a successful fixed price contract is to bid a price that covers both direct and indirect costs."

"That's true," Selman replied. "Our problem is that we don't know what our product costs are. Without a cost accounting system, we have to guess."

Distinguishing Characteristics of Cost Accounting and Financial Accounting

Dr. Flagg, who knew little about finance, interrupted. "What's a cost accounting system?" he asked.

Wycoff, a retired Wall Street banker, looked up from the financial report he was studying. "It's an accounting system that accumulates costs by product." "Prior to the introduction of PPS, cost accounting was almost nonexistent in the healthcare industry."

"How's a cost accounting system different from what we already have?" Flagg asked.

"Our present system—which is a financial accounting system—accumulates costs by department but not by product," Wycoff replied. "It's used primarily for generating financial statements. A cost accounting system would give us data on *individual product* costs. As Selman says, without cost data, accurate pricing is impossible."

Flagg still wasn't certain what Wycoff was talking about. "By products do you mean the services we sell?" Flagg asked.

"The goods and services," Wycoff replied. "Catherization kits, surgical packs, bed baths, tonsillectomies . . ."

Historical Pricing in Hospitals

Helen waited until she was certain Flagg understood Wycoff's explanation. When Flagg nodded, she continued, her dark eyes boring in on Selman.

"You didn't know what your costs were, Mr. Selman? You told me that prior to PPS, you were paid under a cost reimbursement system. How could insurance companies pay you costs if you didn't know what your costs were?"

Flagg liked Ingersol's argument. "Touché!" he said, slapping the table with his cadaverous hand. Satisfied with himself, he beamed at the board. Everyone ignored him.

"Under cost reimbursement," Selman said, "we accumulated costs *per patient day*. There was never an attempt to accumulate costs by *specific product or diagnosis.*"

Helen raised her eyebrows skeptically. "I have trouble believing that's true," Helen said. "Whenever I've had a family member in the hospital, I've received a bill itemizing costs right down to the last $10 aspirin!"

"We had a charge schedule," Selman admitted, "but charges were not always based on costs. Prices were determined by what the competition was charging, or what the market could bear. Overall, we received enough revenue to cover total expenses—but some products subsidized others."

Selman noticed that David Brannan's face was turning red. He continued, doing his best to ignore him. "It wasn't necessary to know the costs of individual products under cost reimbursement," he said. "All we had to know was total cost per patient day. For the Mountainlands prospective payment system contract, we needed more accurate cost data."

Brannan cut him off. "The problem isn't cost accounting!" he shouted. "The problem is management! Management doesn't plan—it spends all of its time putting out fires."

"Actually Mr. Brannan," Selman said, breaking in.

"Don't interrupt me!" Brannan snapped. "The reputation of the hospital is plummeting. Employee morale is low, productivity is lower, and service is rotten. I can't attend Rotary without getting deluged with complaints about service. I'm fed up with it!" he shouted angrily.

Selman waited until Brannan had finished. "All the problems you mention relate to our lack of cost accounting. Without product cost data, it's difficult to do strategic planning—we don't know which lines are profitable and which ones aren't."

"Employee productivity may be a problem," he continued, "but without a cost accounting system, it's been difficult to establish labor standards and impossible to calculate variances. Without variances, you can't tell the efficient departments from the inefficient ones."

"Your third complaint is employee morale. Most of our morale problems have been caused by the uncertainty generated by our losses, which were caused by poor pricing, which, in turn, was caused by the lack of cost accounting data."

Selman turned to Wycoff, who had a better understanding of these matters. "The adoption of a cost accounting system should solve all of those problems," he said.

Wycoff was unimpressed. "Two years ago, the board directed you to install a cost accounting system. You ignored our directive."

"I wasn't given the money to implement it," Selman replied defensively.

"Eighteen months ago, I opposed bidding on the Mountainlands contract without cost data," Wycoff said. "Hap Castleton moved ahead anyway—on your recommendation!"

"If we hadn't bid the contract, we would have lost the business to competitors." Selman replied. "We couldn't afford the drop in volume."

"We'd have been better off not to bid the contract than to absorb the losses it has incurred," Wycoff retorted.

"I don't know if that's true," Selman said. "Most of our costs are fixed. I don't think we could have cut variable costs enough to compensate for the decline in volume."

"That's just the point!" said Wycoff, slamming his fist on the table, "WE DON'T KNOW! And you're the person responsible for providing us the data!"

A few minutes later, Selman was terminated.

Supplement Two

Variance Analysis

From the Journal of Wes Douglas

Today I met with Natalie Simpson, my new acting controller, to formulate a plan to put the hospital at breakeven within ninety days. To reach that objective, we must reduce costs, increase revenues or a combination of both. We decided to focus on costs first.

As we began, Natalie provided me with data from the Utah Healthcare Association showing that labor costs per patient day are higher at Peter Brannan Community Hospital than at most other facilities of comparable size. The obvious question is, *why?*

In trying to formulate an answer, I drew upon my experience as a manufacturing consultant. Two years ago, I conducted a study for Mallory Manufacturing, the company that builds the titanium engine pods for military aircraft. Mallory's customers at that time included Lockheed, McDonnell Douglas, and Boeing. Because both labor and titanium are expensive, Mallory needed a standard cost accounting system that would monitor labor and material costs accurately.

One of the most useful reports of the system I designed for Mallory was the *Labor and Materials Variance Report*. A *variance* is the difference between what something should cost and what it actually costs. For example, the standard number of labor hours to manufacture an engine pod for an F-16 fighter was determined by industrial engineers to be 280 hours. The standard labor rate for those manufacturing the pod was $15.50 per hour. Total standard labor costs for an F-16 pod, therefore, were 280 hours times $15.50 = $4,340. If the actual costs to manufacture an engine pod were $4,500, Mallory Manufacturing would have incurred an unfavorable variance of $4,340 - $4,500 = -$160.

Variances explain the difference between standard (or budgeted cost) and actual cost. An unfavorable labor variance can occur if the firm pays a higher labor rate or uses more labor hours than the standard allows. Labor variances can be broken into rate and efficiency variances, which can be calculated with the following formulas:

Labor Rate Variance:

[Actual Labor Hours x Actual Labor Rate] - [Actual Labor Hours X Standard Labor Rate]
and

Labor Efficiency Variance:

[Actual Labor Hours x Standard Labor Rate] - *[Standard Labor Hours x Standard Labor Rate]*

Natalie called the Utah Healthcare Association to obtain the following information from other hospitals:

Table 1—Nursing Hours Per Patient Day
Utah Healthcare Association Data

	Peter Brannan Community Hospital	Hospital A	Hospital B	Hospital C
Medical	5.4	4.40	3.75	4.00
Surgical	7.1	6.50	4.50	5.10
Obstetric	6.6	5.20	3.90	4.65
Pediatrics	5.1	4.70	3.00	4.10
Average	6.04	5.10	3.81	4.67

A second phone call provided her with a schedule of average labor rates for registered nurses, as shown in Table 2.

Table 2—RN Nursing Cost Per Patient Day
Utah Healthcare Association Data

	Peter Brannan Community Hospital	Hospital A	Hospital B	Hospital C
Medical	$90.45	$57.20	$44.90	$52.50
Surgical	$112.89	$85.05	$54.25	$66.30
Obstetric	$105.60	$68.25	$46.00	$61.45
Pediatrics	$82.11	$61.15	$36.70	$53.20
Average	$97.86	$71.50	$45.50	$58.80

As Natalie and I analyzed Table 2, we found little correlation between Peter Brannan Community Hospital's hourly wage rates for identified positions and those of competing hospitals. Puzzled, we met with Don Yanamura, director of human resources, to determine how these labor rates had been established. To our surprise, we learned that wage rates were set by supervisors without a clear description of what the job incumbent would be doing, or what the market rate was paying for similar jobs.

Consequently, I decided to take a two-pronged approach to the question of determining labor variances.

The first step would be to hire a consultant to assist Yanamura in establishing wage rates that not only would be fair, but would be competitive with those of other hospitals. This would provide *a standard rate* for the labor. The second step would be to develop industrial engineered time motion work sampling labor standards for the services and products provided by the hospital. This would provide me with *standard hours* for labor. Armed with this information, I could then begin to calculate labor variances.

That afternoon, I called Karisa Holyoak who provided me the name of Dr. Irene Cowdrey, a compensation consultant. A preliminary meeting was scheduled with Cowdrey to discuss the scope of a possible compensation.

* * *

"I've never been through a compensation study before," Yanamura said during our subsequent meeting with Dr. Irene Cowdrey. "What information will you need from my staff, and what will be your methodology?"

"We need copies of your present salary schedules, organization charts, and job descriptions."

"Salary schedules and organizational charts are no problem," Yanamura said, "but the few job descriptions we have are outdated."

"Our firm can prepare those," Cowdrey said, "but it will increase your cost.

Yanamura looked at me questioningly. "I don't see that we have a choice." Cowdrey noted the change and then stood and walked to the board. "The study will have ten phases," she said, writing the following:

- *Data gathering*
- *Initial meeting with employees*
- *Preparation of job descriptions*
- *Employee interviews*
- *Identification and rating of job characteristics*
- *Calculation of job points through regression analysis*
- *Selection of benchmark positions and collection of market pay data*
- *Preparation of hospital salary line*
- *Preparation of salary schedule*
- *Final report*

"We've already discussed data gathering," Cowdrey commented, returning the chalk to the tray. Retrieving a handkerchief from her coat, she wiped the chalk dust off her fingers. "Next, we will be meeting with your employees to explain the study, answer any questions, and get them started on their job descriptions. We will provide the format. Employees should prepare the first draft, which should be reviewed and approved by their supervisors before their interview."

"What happens in the interview?" Yanamura asked.

Job Tasks and Job Characteristics

"We start by reviewing job tasks. Then we move directly to an evaluation and numerical rating of job characteristics."

"What are *job characteristics*?" I asked, referencing point five, "And how are they different from job tasks?"

"A *job task* is an activity performed by an employee—like typing a letter or changing a sterile dressing. A *job characteristic* is a *behavior* that must be exhibited by the job incumbent. A good example might be the need to work with numbers, or the supervision of other employees, or meeting with the public."

Cowdrey searched my eyes for a signal that I understood what she was talking about. The expression on my face signaled that I didn't. Cowdrey was quiet for a moment as she thought of other ways to explain the concept.

A History of Job Analysis

"Maybe it would help if I gave a brief history of job analysis," Cowdrey said. "Job analysis is about fifty-five years old. It started in the 1940s, when governmental and business organizations recognized the need to design compensation systems that not only were fair, but could be explained to the average employee.

"The original approach was to list tasks performed by an employee, cluster jobs into broad groups according the similarity of their tasks, and then assign compensation to job groups."

Yanamura was taking notes. "That approach makes sense," he said. "Analyze a job's tasks and you have analyzed the job."

"Initially, that's what the analysts thought," said Cowdrey. "Unfortunately, it didn't work. There are millions of tasks in the world of work—assigning a numerical value to each of them is an impossible assignment."

"What's the alternative?" Yanamura asked.

"The assignment of numerical values to *job characteristics*. In 1976, an industrial psychologist named McCormick developed a structured job questionnaire of what he called 'worker-oriented elements.' He was able to identify 186 elements common to all jobs. These were divided into six divisions." Cowdrey turned to write on the board.

- *Information input*
- *Mental processes*
- *Work output*
- *Relationship with other persons*
- *Job context*
- *Other job characteristics*

"Item one, *information input*, is concerned with the information an employee must have to perform his or her job, and the way he or she gets that information."

"How does a person get information to do his or her job?" Cowdrey asked. Answering her own question, she wrote this on the board:

Information can be obtained by:

- *Reading (manuals, memos, letters, reports)*
- *Listening (speech, sounds, signals)*
- *Observing (gauges, dials, nonverbal facial behaviors)*
- *Touching*
- *Smelling*
- *Sensing*

"McCormick developed a *Position Analysis Questionnaire* that job analysts use to evaluate 186 job characteristics, including the six listed above. Each characteristic is ranked, on a scale of 1 to 5, using a measurement system provided in the questionnaire. For example, one job that doesn't require much reading is that of a crosswalk guard. That position would probably receive a '*one.*' A legal assistant, on the other hand, who does a great deal of reading might receive a '*four*' or '*five.*'"

"Okay—I understand what job characteristics are, and how they are rated, " I said. "What's the next step in the study?"

Regression Analysis

"Calculation of job evaluation points through regression analysis," replied Cowdrey.

"*Regression what?*" asked Yanamura.

"Regression analysis," repeated Cowdrey. Picking up her chalk, she returned to the board. "In high school you probably learned the equation for a straight line," Cowdrey said, writing the following on the board.

Equation One:

$Y = a + bX$

"Graphed, the equation looks something like this," she continued.

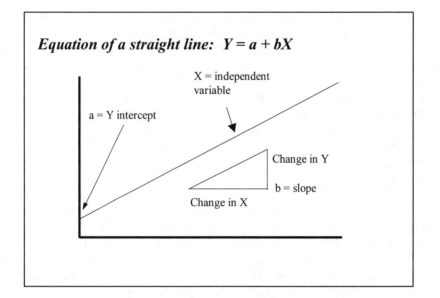

Equation of a straight line: $Y = a + bX$

X = independent variable

a = Y intercept

Change in Y

b = slope

Change in X

"X is the independent variable, Y is the dependent variable, a is a constant represented by the Y intercept, and b, also known as beta, is the slope Y."

Yanamura squinted as he studied the board. "I remember something about that," he mumbled.

"This is also the formula for linear regression," said Cowdrey, "a modeling technique used to establish the relationship between two variables, X and Y.

"Let's use a medical example and assume we're studying the relationship between lung cancer, which we will label as variable Y, and smoking, which we will label as variable X. If the X line has an upward slope, there is a positive correlation—the more you smoke, the greater the chance of developing cancer."

"But we know that more than one thing can cause cancer. How does this model capture that?" asked Yanamura.

"It doesn't; that's why we need multiple regression. Scientists who want to determine the effect of several independent variables on one dependent variable use multiple regression. As you stated, there are many factors that increase the chances that a smoker will get cancer. These are the multiple independent variables. What might these be?" she asked. Yanamura listed the following factors, which Cowdrey wrote on the board.

Variables Affecting the Possibility of Acquiring Cancer:

- *Tobacco use*
- *Alcohol consumption*
- *Fat intake*
- *Fiber intake*
- *Exercise*
- *Age*

"Excellent!" said Cowdrey. "The equation would be:

Equation Two:

$$Y = a + b_1X_1 + b_2X_2 + b_3X_3 + b_4X_4 + b_5X_5 + b_6X_6$$

"Where X_1 was the number of cigarettes smoked daily, X_2 was the ounces of liquor consumed, X_3 was the ounces of fat eaten, etc."

"Are those the *independent variables*?" Yanamura asked.

"Right," Cowdrey replied.

"Then what are the *b*s?"

"The *b*s, or betas, tell how important each independent variable is in increasing the chance of cancer. If b_1, the beta for cigarettes, had a value of 14, while b_2, the beta for alcohol, had a value of 7, then we could conclude that the impact of tobacco on causing cancer was twice that of alcohol."

"How would you calculate Y, the probability of a person's getting cancer, assuming you knew the betas and the X values?" Yanamura asked.

"By multiplying the Xs and the *b*s and summing them," Cowdrey said. "That's what is known as the '*sum of the cross products.*'"

The room was silent for a moment while Yanamura digested this. "Now let's apply multiple regression to the problem of compensation," Cowdrey said. "In the formula developed by McCormick, the Y variable is compensation points. The X variables are the job characteristics that McCormick determined have the greatest influence on pay—we discussed those a moment ago."

"How did McCormick calculate the betas?" Yanamura asked, studying the equation.

"Through the use of matrix algebra to solve the equation for b" Cowdrey replied. "I won't show you how it's done—just trust me that it's possible." Cowdrey returned to the board. "Let's simplify McCormick's model by assuming that there are only three—rather than 187—job characteristics that influence pay. Let's say these are:

- *Number of people supervised*
- *Numbers of years of education*
- *Number of years of experience*

"Let's also assume that the betas as determined by the compensation analyst for each of these factors are as follows: job characteristic number 1 has a beta of 4, job characteristic number 2 has a beta of 6, and job characteristic number 3 has a beta of 3. Let's also assume that the constant is 2. The equation would then be written as follows:"

Equation Three:

$$Y = 2 + 4X_1 + 6X_2 + 3X_3$$

Cowdrey studied the equation for a moment. "Now that we have the equation," she said, "all we have to do is rank the X values for each job. Let's pretend we are evaluating a nursing supervisor. From data provided, we determine that this person supervises 3 people, has 2.5 years of education, and 10.7 years of experience. The equation would now read:

Equation Four:

$$Y = 2 + 4(3) + 6(2.5) + 3(10.7)$$

Or

$$Y = 61.1$$

"The total job points for this person would be 61.1 points," Cowdrey said. "Obviously, with 187 variables rather than three, the model would be more accurate."

Yanamura's eyes lit with understanding. "Okay," he said. "I understand how you calculate job evaluation points for each position; now show me how you use them in establishing labor rates."

I was pleased with Yanamura's understanding and enthusiasm. For our compensation study to succeed, it was essential that our human resource director buy into the methodology behind the study.

"To show you how we use job evaluation points, let's return to the compensation study steps I wrote earlier on the board," Cowdrey said. "Step 7 is to select benchmark positions and graph present pay against job points. Let's assume, for the sake of simplicity, that the hospital only has nine positions, which have been evaluated using our system. Let's also assume the salary data shown in Table 1.

Table 1—Job Characteristics Rates and Present Hourly Rate for Fictional Hospital

1	2	3
Position	Job evaluation points	Present Hourly Rate
Business Office Mgr.	72.0	$17.00
Nurse Supervisor	61.1	$15.20
Acct. Supervisor	60.0	$20.00
Senior Accountant	42.5	$11.35
RN	41.0	$18.00
Materials Clerk	31.2	$14.05
LPN	31.0	$11.00
Nurse Aide	12.0	$10.00
Unit Clerk	12.0	$ 6.20

Cowdrey retrieved two charts from a notebook and handed them to Yanamura. "If we graph present salary against job evaluation points, as I have done in Chart 1, we can see a rough correlation between market and the hospital's present salary program."

"I take it that the line represents the hospital's salary line, as calculated by your regression model," I said.

"That's right," replied Cowdrey. "If the hospital's only concern was internal consistency, the data indicate that the accounting supervisor makes too much—his or her pay should be approximately $17.50. The nurse supervisor makes too little—his or her pay should also be approximately $17.50. The proposed salary schedule is shown as Chart 2."

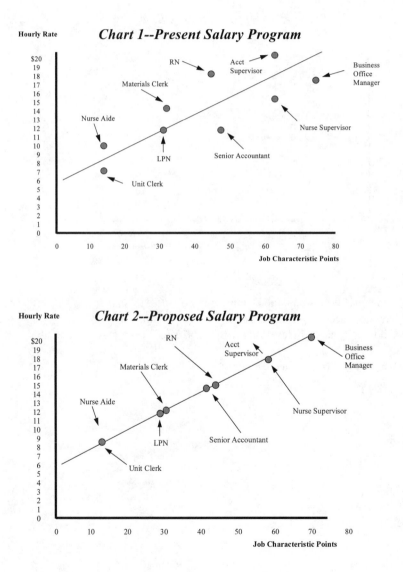

"If the hospital's concern was external consistency, it would want to use industry averages for the data points to determine an industry salary line. This could then be compared with the hospital's salary line to see how the hospital's wages compared with industry. For example, one hospital I worked with had a comparatively flat salary schedule. Lower-paid employees were receiving more money than market, while higher-paid employees were paid less. This was illustrated in the following chart."

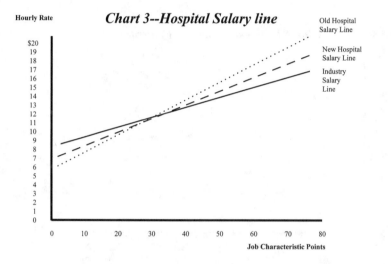

"As a result of the study, the hospital moved closer to market."

"I like the objectivity of the model," said Yanamura.

"So do I," I said. "How long will it take to finish a study like this for our hospital?"

"About six weeks," replied Cowdrey.

"Let's do it."

Supplement Three

Calculating Labor Variances

Wednesday morning, Irene Cowdrey, Natalie Simpson, and Human Resource Director Don Yanamura were back to report their progress in establishing labor standards—the standards that would allow Wes to determine why Peter Brannan Community Hospital's labor costs were higher than those of so many other hospitals.

The discussion initially focused on the definition of the cost centers for which variances would be calculated. Wes defined these cost centers as *primary products and services.* An example of a primary *product* is a dressing change, an injection or a prescription. An example of a primary *service* is a bed bath or the suturing of a wound.

Calculating the Cost of a Primary Product

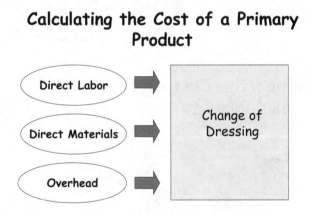

Once standard costs were established for these basic products, they could then be "rolled up" into an intermediate product, such as a major surgical procedure or an emergency center visit.

Calculating the Cost of an
Intermediate Product

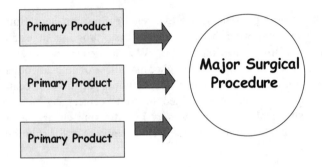

Calculating the Cost of a
Final Product

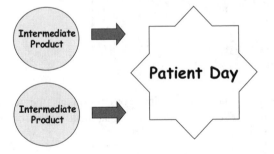

These, in turn, could be rolled into final products, such as DRGs, admissions, capitation days, or patient days.

"Rolling up primary costs to calculate intermediate costs, and intermediate costs to calculate final product costs, makes sense from a theoretical viewpoint," Wes said. "A year from now, I hope that's what we are doing. Right now, however, we don't have time to install a system with that complexity—there are 30,000 primary products in the hospital. In addition, we need the data from Irene Cowdrey's study, which won't be available for several more weeks. In the interim, can't you give me something simpler?"

"We could do a *quick-and-dirty study* to determine the direct labor, direct materials, and overhead components of our first final product, the patient day," Natalie said.

"Quick & Dirty"

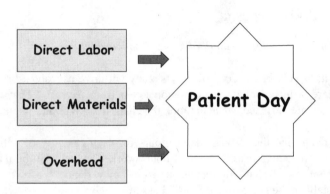

"Eventually," she continued, "when we have more resources, including the Cowdrey data, we can use the more sophisticated methodology to roll up primary and intermediate product costs to a whole host of other final products, including *capitation days, diagnostic related groups*, etc."

"For the time being, however, the product will be defined as a patient day?" asked Wes.

"That's right."

"Sounds like a good temporary solution to me. I suggest one enhancement. Instead of one initial final product, *a patient day*, let's have six product classifications." Wes stood and wrote on the board:

Initial products—quick and dirty system:

- *Medical patient day*
- *Surgical patient day*
- *Obstetrical patient day*
- *Pediatric patient day*
- *Intensive care unit patient day*
- *Nursery patient day*

"That's a good idea," Natalie replied.

"Now lets talk about the calculation of variances for each category of patient day. I want both *labor rate* and *labor efficiency variances,*" Wes said. He walked to the board:

Calculation of Labor Rate Variance:

(actual hours x actual labor rate) – (actual hours x standard labor rate) = labor rate variance

Calculation of Labor Efficiency Variance:

(actual hours x standard labor rate) – (standard hours x standard labor rate)

"We'll give them to you, boss. Dr. Cowdrey's study will give us standard rates, which we will compare with actual rate information taken from payroll. That will allow us to calculate the rate variance." Natalie took the chalk from Wes and wrote the following on the board:

"We'll have to determine the standard labor hours for each category of patient day, of course. These will be compared to actual hours worked, which will be taken from payroll." Yanamura said. "That will give us our efficiency variance."

"How will we establish the standard for time?" I asked.

"There are several approaches," Natalie said. She wrote the following on the board:

Approaches to establishing time standards for labor

- *The hospital can hire an industrial engineer to perform a time and motion work sampling study to establish standard hours*

- *The hospital can borrow standards developed by other hospitals that are about the same size as Peter Brannan Community Hospital.*

- *The hospital can adopt Peter Brannan Community Hospital's historical hours per patient day as its first standard, hoping to tighten those standards as better data becomes available.*

After some discussion, the option chosen was a combination of the last two approaches, and the meeting adjourned.

✻ ✻ ✻

Later that afternoon, Wes Douglas, Natalie Simpson, Don Yanamura, and Irene Cowdrey met with Elizabeth Flannigan, Director of Nursing, who was surprised at the difference in nursing labor cost per patient day between Peter Brannan Community Hospital and that of other facilities of similar size. At first, she resisted establishing efficiency standards for her nurses, feeling that it was another attempt by administration to ratchet nursing workload up.

She consented to the new program, however, when Wes proposed that one-third of the saving arising from the attainment of tighter standards be placed in a bonus pool for distribution on an annual basis to nursing personnel. If the nursing department were able to meet the proposed standard, the total bonus would be in the neighborhood of $531,000.

Supplement Four

Pricing Products and Services

Wes Douglas shook his head as he tore a leaf from the small calendar pad on his desk. It was hard to believe how quickly his time at Peter Brannan Community Hospital had passed. Given the complexity, he took satisfaction in his growing understanding of healthcare finance. Still, there was much to learn; and he grimaced as he contemplated the remaining activities necessary to get his hospital in the black. Having learned from Pete Lister how to increase volume, Wes decided it was now time to address the issue of price.

The following day, he met with Natalie Simpson, who explained how the hospital makes or loses money under the most common payment systems.

Billed Charges

Billed charge systems, Simpson explained, are used for individuals who do not have health insurance and for small insurance companies that cannot negotiate discounts or prospective payment systems. The only way for a hospital to lose money under a billed charge system is to charge less than costs. Studies indicate that many hospitals set billed charges at a level where they will not only recoup the cost of treating the patient but also will subsidize Medicare, Medicaid, and some large insurance companies that pay less than costs.

Cost Plus Reimbursement

Cost reimbursement was the traditional payment system Medicare, Medicaid, and some other insurance companies used. If a hospital makes cost plus 3 percent, the easiest way to increase profits is to let costs increase. You can lose money under cost reimbursement by not knowing the Federal regulations, not knowing your costs, or by poor accounting practices.

DRG Payment

The DRG payment system pays a fixed price per diagnostic related group. Medicare establishes the payment amount for its DRG payment system. To avoid losing money, hospitals must reduce costs below the DRG payment, or not offer the service.

Some insurance companies have instituted their own DRG payment programs. These rates are negotiable. Hospitals must know what their primary, intermediate, and final product costs are if they are to prosper under DRG reimbursement.

Capitation Payment

Capitation payments were negotiated with health insurance companies. The average payment received by PBCH was $30 a month per enrollee. In return for the monthly payment, the hospital agreed to provide all inpatient services for patients admitted under the plan. Under capitation payment, the hospital received its money regardless of whether patients were admitted. It was to the hospital's benefit to keep these patients *out* of the hospital. *An interesting twist,* Wes thought.

To price the capitation payment accurately, the hospital had to estimate the annual cost of each employee group. To do this, it hired an actuary to analyze the demographics of each employer.

Utilization by employee group was of little value without internal cost data. With the *"quick and dirty"* costing system installed by Natalie, cost could be tracked by seven categories of patient day. That detail was not sufficient for capitation payment, however. The system must have the capability to accumulate costs by primary and intermediate product. Natalie summarized her concerns with the capitation payment system by writing the following on the board:

- *We have no experience in working with actuaries to determine estimated volumes by employer group.*

- *We don't have product costs to use in estimating annual cost once we estimate the volume. Without cost data, effective bidding is impossible, as is cost control.*

- *We don't understand all the liabilities associated with capitation payment. In addition, we have little experience in accounting for the insurance products we are being forced to offer.*

When the meeting ended, Wes decided there was little he could do about pricing until he had a viable cost accounting system. He established this as his next priority.

Supplement Five

Information Needs of Managers

Tuesday morning, Wes met with key department heads and physicians to discuss the design and installation of the expanded hospital cost accounting system. To minimize distractions, the meeting was held at Dr. Amos's cabin in Little Cottonwood Canyon.

"I've never been involved with service industry cost accounting," said Wes, as the final participant in the meeting settled into her chair. "The time has come, however, to start designing our new system. To expedite the process, I've decided to form a committee—I'll serve as chair, and beginning this morning, you are all committee members."

"Tell me about your information needs," he continued. "What do you need to run your departments? What information must our expanded cost accounting system provide to you?"

The supervisors were silent for a moment as they thought about his request. The first to speak was Helen Wheeler, business office manager.

Pricing

"I need a cost accounting system for pricing," Helen said. "Insurance companies are increasingly asking us to bid on a fixed price basis."

"Is pricing a high priority?" Wes asked the other supervisors.

"I think it's our first priority," said Natalie Simpson. "The Mountainlands contract is up for renewal. We can't bid that contract unless we have a good handle on our costs."

Cost Control

"What's your second priority?" Wes asked the group.

Natalie raised her hand. "We need a cost accounting system for cost control," she said.

"You're still interested in variance analysis?" Wes asked.

"Yes, although I'm not sure that traditional variances will provide us enough information. In analyzing a labor or material variance, I would like to know something about *acuity of illness*, for example."

"What's that?" Wes asked.

"Acuity refers to severity of illness."

"How do you measure something as ambiguous as that?"

"At the beginning of each shift, our nurses classify each patient on the floor into one of five acuity levels, based on the care they will require for the shift. Factors considered include whether the patient's conscious, if the patient can feed himself, etc. Different levels of acuity require different levels of care."

"It seems as though the classification system would be fairly subjective," Wes said.

Elizabeth was defensive. "We have well-defined criteria. I'll be happy to review them with you if you question what we are doing," she said. Wes noticed the fire in her eyes. This was neither the time nor the place to take on Elizabeth Flannigan.

"I'm sure you have a good system, but sometime I would like to see what you're doing," Wes replied, turning the focus of his attention back to variances.

"To establish product variances, one must first define the product," Wes continued. "At Mallory Manufacturing, our product was engine pods—we produced them for three different aircraft. In a complex service industry like a hospital, it seems that product definition is a vastly more difficult chore. What's our product here at Peter Brannan Community Hospital?"

"That's a good question," replied Elizabeth. "Not many years ago, when hospitals were paid on a cost-reimbursement basis, the basic product was a patient day. From what Natalie told me, Medicare would come in at the end of the year and audit our books to determine our average cost per patient day."

"That's right," replied Natalie. "Using a step-down methodology, auditors would allocate service department costs to revenue-producing departments to determine total department costs. They would then divide this by total patient days to determine the average cost per patient day—it was a simple methodology."

Management PPS Information Needs
• Pricing
• Cost control
• Strategic planning
• Measurement of comparative hospital efficiency

"It may have been simple, but it doesn't sound like it was very accurate," Wes said.

"It wasn't," Natalie acknowledged. "I think the payment system drives the definition of a product in the current environment. Under DRG reimbursement, for example, the product should probably be a diagnostic related group. Presently, there are approximately 500. Under a capitation payment system, the product is probably an enrollee month for a specific demographic category. For that calculation, we'll need an actuary."

"It is obvious that our system will have to be flexible enough to accommodate multiple product definitions. How do we accomplish that?" Wes asked.

"By establishing standard costs for primary products and then summarizing or rolling those costs into intermediate products and finally into final products such as the DRG," Natalie said.

"Okay," Wes said. "What other information needs must our expanded system accommodate?"

Strategic Planning

"The board needs a cost accounting system to help with *strategic planning*," volunteered Dr. Amos, "something that can help us understand which product lines are profitable and which are not."

"Give me an example," Wes said.

"With our low volume, I suspect we lose money on inpatient psychiatry and obstetrics," said Amos. "I believe our competition is losing money on their emergency center. If we were sure of our costs, we might approach them with the proposition that *you close your emergency center and give us those patients, and we'll close psychiatry and obstetrics and give you our patients*."

"Strategic planning," Wes said. "Anything else we need from our new cost accounting system?"

Measurement of Comparative Efficiency

"I need some way to compare the efficiency of our nursing department with those of other hospitals in the state," said Elizabeth Flannigan. "You told me that in manufacturing, product cost is often used as a surrogate or substitute for efficiency. If quality is held constant, the most efficient producers will have the lowest per-unit costs. In the health industry, however, per-unit cost is not always a good indicator of efficiency."

"Why not?"

"Because of something we call *'case-mix,'*" Elizabeth replied.

"What's that?" Wes asked.

"Case-mix refers to the complexity of the average case seen in the hospital. The University Hospital, for example, treats more complex cases than we do. It would not be fair to compare the average cost of a patient day at the University Hospital with our average cost."

"What's the solution?"

"We'll have to work on it," Natalie interjected.

Supplement Six

Cost Accounting Taxonomies

That afternoon, the group continued the discussion. Natalie brought her laptop computer and projection equipment to display her data from the computer.

Job Order and Process Costing

"This morning we must decide whether we will install a job-order or process-cost accounting system," Natalie said as the meeting began.

"Tell me the difference," said Elizabeth.

"Companies that manufacture *unique* products use job-order cost systems," Natalie said. "A builder of custom homes, for example, would usually use job-order costing. In a job-order costing system, the costs of direct labor, direct materials, and factory overhead are *accumulated by job*, typically on a job ticket.

"On the other hand, companies that manufacture *homogeneous* products use process-costing systems. Examples include firms that manufacture paint or petroleum. In a process-costing system, the costs of direct labor, direct material, and factory overhead are *accumulated by department* for a period of time. These costs are then divided by units manufactured during the period to determine *unit cost.*"

Since each patient is unique, but some products are homogeneous, Wes opted for a combination of process and job costing.

Actual, Normal, and Standard Cost Systems

"Earlier, we decided we would go with a standard cost system. While I think that decision should stand, it is good to understand the alternatives. Alternatives to a standard cost system include *actual cost accounting* systems and *normal cost accounting* systems," Natalie said.

"In both process- and

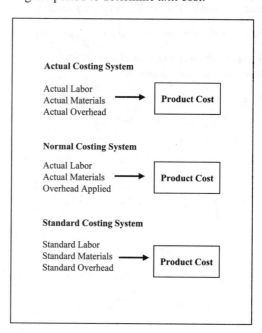

job-order cost accounting systems, manufacturing costs are accumulated in work-in-process accounts. In an actual cost accounting system, the work-in-process account is charged with *actual direct labor, actual direct materials, and actual factory overhead.* Few companies use actual cost accounting systems because it may result in inequitable allocations of factory overhead. If a company incurs more factory utilities in the winter months, for example, it doesn't make sense to charge products manufactured during this season with more overhead.

"For this reason, many companies use *normal cost accounting* systems. In a normal cost accounting system, work-in-process is charged with actual direct labor and actual direct materials. Overhead is allocated to production based on a normal or average rate.

"*Standard cost accounting* systems, the type we have selected, charge work-in-process with *standard direct labor and standard direct materials.* Overhead is charged at a *standard factory overhead rate.*"

"What are the advantages of standard cost accounting?" Elizabeth asked.

Natalie returned to the board where she wrote the following:

Standard Costing will allow:

• *More accurate information on the reasons we are making or losing money on individual products.*

• *Variance information on labor, materials, and overhead.*

• *An easier methodology for assigning costs to individual products. Tracking actual costs by patient for 30,000 primary products is not currently feasible.*

• *Better cash planning and inventory control.*

• *A way to involve employees in cost cutting measures through incentive bonuses if new labor standards are met.*

• *A better methodology for the implementation of responsibility accounting.*

Supplement Seven

Designing Accounting Reports to Match Information Needs

"Earlier, we talked about the different types of prospective payment contracts," said Elizabeth Flannigan. "The hospital makes or loses money in different ways under each contract. How will you determine what information to include on each report? My people are tired of getting reports that are so general they are useless for making decisions."

"I suggest we identify report content by asking the following questions," Wes said. As Wes spoke, Natalie wrote the following on the board:

Questions to ask in designing a management accounting report:

- *How does the hospital make or lose money on each contract?*
- *What variables must the supervisor monitor?*
- *What information must be sent on these variables?*
- *How will we gather the information to send the information?*
- *What format should the information take?*
- *How timely must the information be?*

"Let's try this approach on capitation payment," said Natalie. For the next twenty minutes, the group discussed the information that management reports must contain to manage capitation contracts. Natalie led the discussion, serving as scribe at the board. Her finished outline is shown below.

Outline

1) *How do we lose money under a capitation contract?*

   a) *Unnecessary hospital admissions*

   b) *Unnecessary hospital days during necessary hospital stay*

   c) *Treatment of patients in the hospital that could be treated on an outpatient basis*

   d) *Failure to keep patients well through preventive medicine*

   e) *Failure to prevent or reduce nosocomial infections and accidents*

   f) *Failure to detect disease early enough to prevent hospitalization*

g) *Failure to establish premiums that cover the actual cost of treatment*

h) *Not enough information about each program enrollee (age, sex, occupation, medical history)*

i) *Not enough information on expected levels of use by enrollee*

j) *Failure to capture actual cost by patient, by employer, by diagnosis*

2) *What variables must management monitor to prevent losses under capitation payment?*

   a) *The amount and type of preventive medicine provided by plan physicians and hospitals*

   b) *The number and kind of cases treated on an inpatient and on an outpatient basis*

   c) *The average time to detect treatable disease.*

   d) *The average length of hospital stay by diagnosis*

   e) *Population morbidity and mortality rates*

3) *What signals must accounting send on these variables?*

   a) *Selected diagnostic tests per 1,000 enrollees by age and gender*

   b) *Well care visits per 1,000 enrollees by age and gender*

   c) *Number of hospital admissions and patient days per 1,000 enrollees sorted by age, gender, diagnostic category, employer group, occupational category and insurance company*

   d) *Hospital resources consumed sorted by patient, by diagnosis, by age, by sex, but employer groups and occupational class*

4) *Where will accounting get the information to send these signals?*

   a) *Medical records*

   b) *Business office*

   c) *Physicians office*

   d) *Accounting*

   e) *Hospital actuary*

5) *What format should the reports take?*

6) *How timely must the reports be?*

"I think it has been helpful to show how we'll identify the information that our costing system will have to report on each contract type," Natalie said, as she finished writing the list. "Before we get too carried away with detail, however, I would like to talk a little more globally about the purposes the system will serve. Most hospital cost accounting systems perform five functions. Let me write them on the board."

- *Cost determination*
- *Activity forecasting*
- *Functional cost center budgeting*
- *Performance reporting on a product level*
- *Performance reporting on a functional level*

"I recommend," Natalie continued, "that each function become a module in the final cost accounting software program."

Supplement Eight

Designing the Pricing Module

"I'm concerned about the complexity of bringing the entire system up at one time," Wes said as Natalie returned to her seat. "We must learn to walk before we can run."

Wes had been told horror stories of hospitals spending a million dollars or more to implement cost accounting. "We don't have that kind of money, nor the time a system that size takes to install. Are there modules that might meet our immediate needs that could be installed quickly, leaving the design and installation of other modules for a later date?"

"I wondered the same thing," said Natalie. "At an earlier department head meeting, we were told that we need a cost accounting system to support the following four activities." She wrote on the board:

- *Pricing*
- *Cost Control*
- *Strategic Planning*
- *Measurement of Comparative Efficiency*

"We were also told that pricing is our most pressing need," she continued.

"That's true," Wes replied. "The Mountainlands contract is due for renewal."

"A cost accounting system to support pricing decisions is a simpler system than one for cost control," Natalie continued. "Focusing on pricing would simplify the initial system."

"What modules would we need for pricing?" Wes asked, referencing the list of modules Natalie was writing on the board.

- *Cost determination*
- *Activity forecasting*
- *Functional cost center budgeting*
- *Performance reporting on a product level*
- *Performance reporting on a functional level*

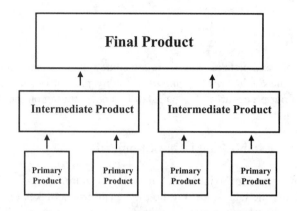

"For pricing, all we need is module one—*cost determination*. The nice thing about module one is that it can be modeled on a PC computer using spreadsheet software."

"That sounds like a good idea," Wes said. "Let's take a ten-minute break. When we return, we'll discuss the components of the cost determination module."

* * *

The sky was the color of gray flannel and large flakes of snow, heavy with moisture, were beginning to fall as the group reconvened in the living room of Amos's cabin. During lunch, Amos had built a fire in the large stone fireplace, and the affable smell of burning pine and hot chocolate filled the cabin.

As Wes stood admiring the granite cliffs of Little Cottonwood Canyon from a large picture window opposite the fireplace, he was pleased with the progress the group had made. Given the hospital's financial situation and the limited experience of the staff in working with cost accounting data, narrowing the focus of the initial costing system to pricing for bidding on prospective contracts seemed like a good idea

Natalie Simpson began the discussion. "In developing standard costs," she said, "Wes and I feel we will probably want to limit ourselves to three levels of detail. The first we'll define as *primary costs*. These are the most basic procedures, services, and products. Examples include a dressing change, a laboratory or radiology test, a physical therapy treatment, or a bed bath.

"The standard costs for primary products are *rolled up* to determine the costs of intermediate products. An intermediate product would include a major surgical procedure like an appendectomy. Standard costs for intermediate products are rolled up to determine the cost of final products such as DRGs, patient days, admissions, or capitation payment enrollee populations.

"Establishing standards for the thousands of primary, secondary, and final products sounds like a lot of work," Elizabeth Flannigan cautioned. "Won't this take years to complete?"

Eighty/Twenty Rule

"It's a big job," said Natalie, "but there are some things we can do to simplify it. The first is to use the *80/20 Pareto principle*. Eighty percent of our revenues come from 20 percent of our procedures. We can start by concentrating on the standard costs of that 20 percent first."

Methodologies for Establishing Labor Standards

"How do you determine the labor cost of each procedure?" responded Elizabeth.

"By determining the labor rate and the time each product takes to produce. The labor rate has already been established through the study conducted by Dr. Irene Cowdrey. To determine standard times, we have several options," said Natalie. "The most accurate would be to determine these through industrially engineered studies."

"Is that where you have a time and efficiency expert follow an employee around to determine how long it takes to perform each activity?" Wes asked.

"That's the methodology," said Natalie.

"We performed some industrial engineering studies at Mallory Manufacturing," Wes said. "They were not only time-consuming but costly. I'm not sure we can afford that approach."

"A second approach would be to borrow standards from other hospitals," said Natalie. "Maybe we could get the University Hospital to share its standards with us."

"The problem with that is University Hospital sees a different type of patient than we do," said Elizabeth. "That hospital's also newer. Our design makes us less cost efficient. It takes more labor to do a procedure here than it would at a more modern facility."

"Why?" Wes asked.

"For one thing, we are crowded," said Elizabeth. "Our employees are literally tripping over each other. That reduces productivity."

Dr. Amos agreed. "Many of our departments weren't designed for current technology," he said. "When our radiology department was built, most of the equipment we use today wasn't invented. We have equipment in the halls and in closets that could be used more effectively if the working areas were designed for the way we do business now."

"Okay, borrowing standards from another hospital is probably out," Wes said glumly.

"We know what our total labor costs for each hospital department are," said Elizabeth. "We also know how many procedures we are performing. Can't we use that data to back into the cost of each procedure?"

"If each procedure took the same time, that would probably work," said Natalie. "We could divide total direct labor costs by total procedures to give us the labor cost per procedure. However, we don't have a homogeneous work unit."

"Actually, many of our professional departments do have a homogeneous work unit; it's called a *relative value unit* or *RVU,*" said Elizabeth.

Natalie's face lit with recognition. "That's right," she said. "The American College of Pathologists, for example, has developed an RVU system for laboratories."

"The radiologists and nurses have done the same thing for their own fields," said Elizabeth.

Relative Value Units (RVUs)

"What's a relative value unit?" Wes asked.

"It's a unit of measure," said Elizabeth. "Though we don't know the exact time it should take a particular hospital to perform a urinalysis or white blood count, there are studies indicating that relative times to perform these two tests are fairly constant. The ratio shouldn't change from hospital to hospital."

Natalie interrupted. "A test with an RVU of 2 should, in theory, take twice as long to perform as a test with an RVU of 1."

"That's right," Elizabeth said.

"If we know the number of relative value units currently performed by each of our professional departments and if we know our variable labor costs, then we should be able to back into a standard labor cost per procedure," Natalie replied.

Isolating Fixed and Variable Labor Costs Through Regression Analysis

"But I see one problem with that," Natalie said, scowling with concern. "We don't know what our variable costs are by department."

"Sure we do," Wes said. "Payroll is processed by department."

"But department payroll costs include *fixed* and *variable* costs," Natalie replied.

"Can't you assume that most of your direct labor costs in a professional department are variable costs, and that most of your overhead labor costs are fixed costs?" Wes asked.

"We could probably make that simplifying assumption," said Natalie. "But I'm not sure how accurate that would be. Some employees are working supervisors; we would have to separate the fixed and variable portions of their pay."

Wes was silent for a moment as he grappled with the problem. Wes knew a controller for a manufacturing company that had wrestled with the same issue. "There's a statistical technique called regression analysis," he said. "It can be used to separate fixed and variable labor costs."

"Of course!" said Natalie. "The spreadsheet program on my computer has a regression analysis program. Give me a few minutes and I'll prepare an example for you."

"Let's take a break," Wes said, "while Natalie builds a regression model on his computer for us to review."

Supplement Nine

Regressing RVUs to Determine Fixed and Variable Costs

While Wes prepared the room for Natalie's presentation, Natalie retrieved a statistical model of a simple hospital that she had created for a demonstration before the meeting. The facility had three service departments—administration, housekeeping, and laundry—and five revenue producing departments—nursing, laboratory (Lab), x-ray, physical therapy (P.T.), and operating room (O.R.).

Each revenue department in the model performed only three procedures. Relative value units for each of the procedures in each of the departments is listed in Table 1.

Table 1
Relative Value Units (RVU) Per Procedure

	Nursing	Lab	X-ray	P.T.	O.R.
Procedure 1	1	2	2	3	1
Procedure 2	3	1	5	4	2
Procedure 3	4	3	3	5	· 3

Table 2
Number of Procedures

	Nursing	Lab	X-ray	P.T.	O.R.
Procedure 1	8,000	14,000	5,000	1,000	100,000
Procedure 2	4,000	6,000	6,000	2,000	120,000
Procedure 3	2,000	5,000	1,000	3,000	110,000
Total	14,000	25,000	12,000	6,000	330,000

Table 1 was created to show the actual number of procedures performed in 1998 for each of the departments in the model hospital. Table 3 was created to show the actual relative value units per month for the year 1998.

Table 3
Total Relative Value Units Per Month 1998

	Nursing	Lab	X-ray	P.T.	O.R.
Jan	2,240	3,920	3,440	2,000	53,600
Feb	2,240	3,920	3,440	2,000	53,600
Mar	2,800	4,900	4,300	2,500	67,000
Apr	2,520	4,410	3,870	2,250	60,300
May	2,520	4,410	3,870	2,250	60,300
Jun	1,960	3,430	3,010	1,750	46,900
Jul	2,240	3,920	3,440	2,000	53,600
Aug	1,680	2,940	2,580	1,500	40,200
Sep	3,080	5,390	4,730	2,750	73,700
Oct	2,520	4,410	3,870	2,250	60,300
Nov	1,680	2,940	2,580	1,500	40,200
Dec	2,520	4,410	3,870	2,250	60,300
Total	28,000	49,000	43,000	25,000	670,000

Note: The 28,000 RVUs for Nursing for the year of 1998 ties to figures shown in Table 1 and Table 2. To verify, multiply the RVUs for each procedure by the total number of procedures for that year. (8,000 x 1) + (4,000 x 3) + (2,000 x 4) = 28,000.

Natalie created Table 4 to show total labor costs for each of the revenue departments in 1998. In creating Tables 2, 3, and 4, Natalie modified actual data taken from Peter Brannan Community Hospital.

Table 4
Actual Labor Spent

	Nursing	Lab	X-ray	P.T.	O.R.
Jan	$1,212,000	$297,040	$351,600	$170,000	$328,000
Feb	$1,212,000	$297,040	$351,600	$170,000	$328,000
Mar	$1,240,000	$308,800	$364,500	$175,000	$395,000
April	$1,226,000	$302,920	$358,050	$172,500	$361,500
May	$1,226,000	$302,920	$358,050	$172,500	$361,500
Jun	$1,198,000	$291,160	$345,150	$167,500	$294,500
July	$1,212,000	$297,040	$351,600	$170,000	$328,000
Aug	$1,184,000	$285,280	$338,700	$165,000	$261,000
Sept	$1,254,000	$314,680	$370,950	$177,500	$428,500
Oct	$1,226,000	$302,920	$358,050	$172,500	$361,500
Nov	$1,184,000	$285,280	$338,700	$165,000	$261,000
Dec	$1,226,000	$302,920	$358,050	$172,500	$361,500
Total	$14,600,000	$3,588,000	$4,245,000	$2,050,000	$4,070,000

When the group reassembled, Natalie spoke. "During the break, I prepared an example of the use of regression analysis to break total costs into fixed and variable components," she said. Let me show you how it works. In college, we learned the equation for a straight line," she said, writing the following on the board:

$Y = a + bX$

"We also learned that the equation could be graphed like this:"

Graph of a Straight Line

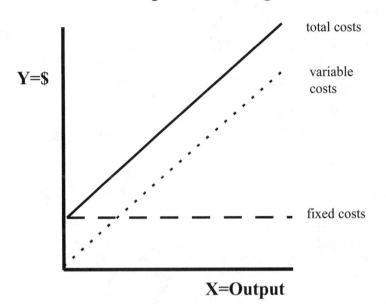

Y=$

total costs

variable costs

fixed costs

X=Output

"The Y variable," she said, pointing to the screen, "is the dependent variable. The X variable is the independent variable; a is the Y-intercept, and b is the slope of the line."

"In a manufacturing setting, this equation is sometimes used to show the relationship between production volume and manufacturing costs. If we adapt this model to our labor costs in the nursing, the Y-axis would represent total labor dollars; the X-axis would represent number of procedure RVUs performed; the a-intercept would represent fixed costs; and the slope, denoted by b, would represent the variable cost per RVU."

"If fixed labor costs in the department were $1,100,000 per month, as is the case in Nursing, and the variable labor costs were $50 per RVU, then the total cost equation for laboratory would be written Y = $1,100,000 + 50x.

"Knowing the equation for any level of production represented by X, we can determine total costs as represented by Y. For example, if we anticipated RVUs, our variable budget would consist of $1,100,000 of fixed costs plus $100,000 of variable costs for a total monthly labor cost of $1,200,000."

"That's fine and well," said Elizabeth. "But how do you calculate the equation? How do you determine that fixed costs are $1,100,000 and variable costs are $50 per relative value unit?"

"Most spreadsheet packages have a regression package that will allow you to calculate a and b if you know X and Y," said Natalie. "I'll show you how it's done.

Table 3 provides our X values—the nursing RVUs. Table 4 provides our Y values—total labor costs. Using Excel software, let's run the equation for nursing. The output from the regression package is shown below:

SUMMARY OUTPUT

Regression Statistics

Multiple R	1
R Square	1
Adjusted R Square	1
Standard Error	2.32831E-10
Observations	12

ANOVA

	df
Regression	1
Residual	10
Total	11

	Coefficients
Intercept	1100000
X Variable 1	50

The Intercept is the monthly fixed costs (1,100,000), and the X Variable 1 is the variable cost per unit (50). We can use the variable cost as the standard labor cost per RVU.

"Give me an example," said Elizabeth.

"Procedure 2 in nursing is worth 3 relative value units. We get that from Table 1. If one RVU worth of labor is worth $50, then a procedure with 3 relative units will be worth $150. That becomes our standard for variable labor for Procedure 1 in the nursing department."

"That's a slick way of coming up with standard costs," said Elizabeth. "Is it as accurate as an industrial engineered study?"

"Probably not," said Natalie, "but it does tell us what our existing standard is. If RVUs are accurate, it should be close."

After studying the data for a moment, Wes spoke. "What I would like to do is use this methodology to calculate standards for the 20 percent of our procedures that generate 80 percent of our revenues. That will give us data that will be good enough for pricing."

"What about those procedures that generate only 20 percent of our revenue?" asked Elizabeth. "How will we establish standard costs for those?"

"Some hospitals use ratio of costs to charges (RCC)," Natalie replied. "It's not accurate, but it's easy to calculate. Accuracy is not that important on a procedure that costs $25 and is produced twice a year. I'll show you how RCC is calculated later," he assured her. "Now, let me run the regression equation for all the departments in our model hospital," she suggested as she performed the calculation and projected the results on the screen as Table 5.

Table 5
Fixed and Variable Costs of Each Revenue Producing Department From Regression

	Nursing	Lab	X-ray	P.T.	O.R.
Fixed	$1,100,000	$250,000	$300,000	$150,000	$200,000
Variable	$50	$12	$15	$10	$5

"As you can see from the table, fixed costs for Nursing are $1,100,000. Variable costs per RVU are $50. By combining these data with those shown in Table 1, we can determine the standard labor costs per procedure. Remember," she said, "the procedure is our *intermediate product*, the building block for our *final product,* the DRG."

"Once again, show us how you do it," said Dr. Amos. "Calculate the standard labor costs for all tests and procedures shown on Table 1."

"Okay," said Natalie as she performed the calculations on her computer and projected them on the screen as Table 6.

Table 6
Direct Labor Cost Per Procedure

	Nursing	Lab	X-ray	P.T.	O.R.
Procedure 1	$ 50	$24	$30	$30	$ 5
Procedure 2	$150	$12	$75	$40	$10
Procedure 3	$200	$36	$45	$50	$15

Supplement Ten

Direct Materials and Hospital Overhead

"Now that we have direct labor costs for each procedure, how do we calculate direct material cost?" asked Elizabeth.

"That's easy," said Natalie. "We pull invoices to determine the materials that go into each test or procedure. Let me make up some data to show how the model works. I'll title it Table 1."

Table 1
Direct Material Cost Per Procedure

	Nursing	Lab	X-ray	P.T.	O.R.
Procedure 1	$34	$12	$12	$4	$3
Procedure 2	$85	$16	$34	$2	$4
Procedure 3	$180	$52	$55	$9	$7

Standard Overhead per Unit of Production
Two General Classes of Overhead

"Our next step is the application of overhead," said Natalie when the table was finished. "At Peter Brannan Community Hospital, we have two general classes of hospital overhead—*department* overhead and *general hospital* overhead. Department overhead includes the indirect costs of the department. In nursing, for example, it includes the salary of Elizabeth Flannigan and her assistant nursing director. It also includes the cost of department travel, copy machines, telephones, etc."

"What's general hospital overhead?" Wes asked.

"That includes the cost of service departments. Examples include administration, human resources, the business office, medical records, and housekeeping."

"How do we allocate these costs to products?" Wes asked.

Allocating Department Overhead to Units of Production

"We allocate department overhead to products by dividing overhead by the department's total yearly relative value units. That gives a department overhead rate using RVUs as the base. We then multiply this rate by the number of relative value units in each procedure."

"Let's model it," Wes replied.

"Okay," said Natalie, as she divided total department fixed overhead by total department relative units and projected the results on the screen as Table 2. "For simplicity, we'll assume that all fixed costs are overhead costs. In the real world, we could use regression to separate fixed and variable materials etc., but let's keep this model simple."

Table 2
Department Fixed Costs Per RVU

Nursing	Lab	X-ray	P.T.	O.R.
$39.2857	$5.1020	$6.9767	$6.0000	$0.2985

"Our next step is to allocate this cost based on RVUs to individual procedures. These data are shown in Table 3."

Table 3
Department Fixed Costs Per Procedure

	Nursing	Lab	X-ray	P.T.	O.R.
Procedure 1	$39.28571	$10.20408	$13.95349	$18.00000	$0.29851
Procedure 2	$117.85714	$5.10204	$34.88372	$24.00000	$0.59701
Procedure 3	$157.14286	$15.30612	$20.93023	$30.00000	$0.89552

Allocating General Hospital Overhead to Revenue Departments, Then to Units of Production

"The next issue to be addressed," continued Natalie, "is how to determine how much general hospital overhead to distribute to each revenue department and then to each procedure. Remember, we are developing the initial system for pricing, and we must include indirect costs. Later, when we use the system to perform cost-profit-volume analysis, we'll be concerned only about contribution margins—the price of the procedure less the variable cost, which we have defined as direct labor and direct materials."

"Let's start with the allocation of general hospital overhead to revenue departments," Wes said.

Natalie stood up and moved to the board. "As far as methodology is concerned, we have several options," she began as she wrote on the board.

- *The direct method*[8]
- *The step-down method*
- *The reciprocal method*
- *The double apportionment method*

---

[8] For a review of each of these methods, see any introductory managerial accounting textbook.

"Which do you propose?" asked Elizabeth.

"I like the *double apportionment* method. It's more accurate than the step-down method and almost as accurate as the reciprocal method. Its major advantage is that it's easy to set up with spreadsheet software."

Natalie returned to the computer to model the double apportionment allocation method. "Unlike the step-down method," she continued, "the double apportionment method allocates costs to *every* department during the first apportionment. The second apportionment is a simple step-down. The remaining balance in each department is closed to all departments in columns on the worksheet *to the right* of that department. Let me demonstrate it," she said as she punched in data for use in modeling this allocation system. "Table 4," she said, "lists the costs and statistics needed for the double apportionment allocation."

Table 4
Service Department Cost and Hospital Statistics for Double Apportionment

	Administration	Housekeeping	Laundry	Nursing	Lab	X-ray	P.T	O.R.
Costs	$230,000	$300,000	$32,000					
Human Resources	3	8	6	50	7	6	3	11
Square feet	800	400	2,000	25,000	1,800	2,100	3,000	4,000
Pounds of Laundry	100	1,200	200	18,000	500	1,000	2,400	4,000

"Table 5 gives the overhead rates used in steps one and two of the apportionment," she said. "Table 6 is the actual apportionment."

Table 5
Overhead Allocation Rates

First Allocation	
Administration	$2,527.47253
Housekeeping	$8.27441
Laundry	$2.34241
Second Allocation	
Administration	$75.31617
Housekeeping	$0.09006
Laundry	$0.02440

Table 6
Double Apportionment of Service Department Costs to Revenue Producing Department

	Administration	Housekeeping	Laundry	Nursing	Lab	X-ray	Physical Therapy	Operating Room	Total
Costs	$230,000	$300,000	$32,000						$562,000
Allocate Administration	($230,000)	$20,220	$15,165	$126,374	$17,692	$15,165	$7,582	$27,802	($0)
Allocate Housekeeping	$6,620	($320,220)	$16,549	$206,860	$14,894	$17,376	$24,823	$33,098	($0)
Allocate Laundry	$234	$2,811	($63,714)	$42,163	$1,171	$2,342	$5,622	$9,370	$0
Subtotal	$6,854	$2,811	$0	$375,397	$33,757	$34,884	$38,027	$70,270	$562,000
Allocate Administration	($6,854)	$603	$452	$3,766	$527	$452	$226	$828	$0
Allocate Housekeeping		($3,413)	$180	$2,252	$162	$189	$270	$360	($0)
Allocate Laundry			($632)	$439	$12	$24	$59	$98	($0)
Subtotal	($6,854)	($2,811)	$0	$6,457	$702	$665	$555	$1,286	($0)
Total	$0	$0	$0	$381,854	$34,459	$35,549	$38,582	$71,556	$562,000

214

"What we have done," said Natalie, "is to allocate service department costs to revenue producing departments, based on the use of services, as determined by core statistics. The $71,566 shown in the last row of the O.R. column represents general overhead allocated to that department from general hospital overhead. To allocate that to individual products, we first calculate allocated service department costs by RVU as shown in Table 7."

Table 7
Allocated Service Department Costs Per RVU

Nursing	Lab	X-ray	P.T.	O.R.
$13.6376	$0.7032	$0.8267	$1.5433	$0.1068

"Next we allocate these costs to procedures, based on the RVUs per procedure, given earlier. That data we can show in Table 8," Natalie said, as she entered additional data in her computer.

Table 8
Allocated Service Department Costs Per Procedure

	Nursing	Lab	X-ray	Physical Therapy	Operating Room
Procedure 1	$13.63764	$1.40649	$1.65344	$4.62986	$0.10680
Procedure 2	$40.91293	$0.70324	$4.13360	$6.17315	$0.21360
Procedure 3	$54.55058	$2.10973	$2.48016	$7.71643	$0.32040

Review of Process to Establish Standard Costs Per Unit of Production

"Just to review where we have been," said Natalie, "we used regression analysis to divide fixed and variable costs. We used relative value units to back into standard direct labor cost per RVU, and then spread these costs to procedures based on the number of RVUs in each procedure. We then reviewed invoices to determine direct material costs. Next, we allocated fixed department costs to procedures based on RVUs, allocated general overhead costs from service departments to revenue departments using a double apportionment method, and then allocated these costs to procedures based on RVUs."

"Now comes the final step in determining total standard costs for each procedure in our model hospital. We add up the standard costs for direct labor, direct materials, department overhead, and general hospital allocated overhead for each procedure. She entered the data into her laptop computer. There," she said, "I've got it!"

Table 9
Standard Costs per Procedure

	Nursing	Lab	X-ray	P.T.	O.R.
Procedure 1	$136.93	$47.61	$57.60	$56.63	$8.41
Procedure 2	$393.77	$33.80	$148.01	$72.17	$14.81
Procedure 3	$591.69	$105.42	$123.41	$96.72	$23.22

"Let me see if I understand the significance of the data," said Wes as he reviewed the numbers on the screen. "In Laboratory, the standard cost for Procedure 1, which I assume would be a lab test, is approximately $35.61. These are loaded costs, as I understand them—they include department and general hospital overhead."

"That's correct," Natalie confirmed.

Supplement Eleven

Ratio of Cost to Charges (RCC)

The next morning, Wes again met with the staff at Dr. Amos's cabin to continue with the conceptual design of the hospital's first cost accounting system.

"Wes has asked me to review an alternate methodology for the establishment of standard costs," Natalie began. "It's called ratio of costs to charges (RCC). It is not very accurate but because it is still used by some hospitals, let me show you how it works," she said, moving to the board. "These are the steps in an RCC calculation." She wrote:

RCC Methodology

- *Calculate total department costs including allocated overhead.*
- *Calculate total department charges.*
- *Divide department costs by department charges to determine the ratio of costs to charges.*
- *Multiply procedure prices by the ratio of costs to charges to calculate an estimate of procedure costs.*

"Let's model this methodology. Table 1 lists our actual costs, as determined by the RVU methodology. Table 2 lists current charges for all procedures. Again, the basic data were taken from our own hospital; all procedures aren't listed, however, to simplify the model."

Table 1
Standard Costs as Determined by RVU Methodology

	Nursing	Lab	X-ray	Physical Therapy	Operating Room
Procedure 1	$136.92336	$35.61057	$42.60693	$36.62986	$8.40531
Procedure 2	$243.77008	$21.80529	$73.01732	$32.17315	$4.81061
Procedure 3	$391.69344	$69.41586	$78.41039	$46.71643	$8.21592

Table 2
Current Charges Before Discovery of Actual Costs

	Nursing	Lab	X-ray	P.T.	O.R.
Procedure 1	$500	$40	·$40	$75	$15
Procedure 2	$600	$55	$190	$105	$15
Procedure 3	$800	$120	$150	$120	$15

"Multiplying actual costs per procedure times the actual number of procedures performed during the year gives us *total costs* for the year, by department. We will call this Table 3. In the real world, we would get this information from the department income statement. However, since I want the model to be consistent, we'll use this methodology to determine department costs."

Table 3
Total Department Costs

	Nursing	Lab	X-ray	P.T.	O.R.	Total
Procedure 1	$1,095,387	$666,548	$228,035	$56,630	$840,531	$2,947,130
Procedure 2	$1,575,080	$202,832	$888,104	$216,519	$1,777,274	$4,659,809
Procedure 3	$1,183,387	$527,079	$123,410	$193,433	$2,553,751	$4,581,061
Total	$3,853,854	$1,396,459	$1,299,549	$466,582	$5,171,556	$12,188,000

"Department charges per product are multiplied by actual numbers of procedures performed to determine revenue by department. Again, in the real world, we would go to the income statement to get this information."

Table 4
Total Department Charges for 1995

	Nursing	Lab	X-ray	P.T.	O.R.	Total
Procedure 1	$4,000,000	$560,000	$200,000	$75,000	$1,500,000	$6,335,000
Procedure 2	$2,400,000	$330,000	$1,140,000	$315,000	$1,800,000	$5,985,000
Procedure 3	$1,600,000	$600,000	$150,000	$240,000	$1,650,000	$4,240,000
Total	$8,000,000	$1,490,000	$1,490,000	$630,000	$4,950,000	$16,560,000

"The ratio of cost to charges for each department is shown below in Table 5."

Table 5
Department Ratio of costs to charges (RCC)

Nursing	Lab	X-ray	P.T.	O.R.
.481731757	0.9372208	0.872180504	0.740606598	1.044758757

Note: The .481731757 figure shown for Nursing is calculated by dividing total nursing costs of $3,853,854 by total nursing revenues of $8,000,000.

"To calculate standard costs using the RCC methodology, multiply individual department charges by the ratio of costs to charges."

Table 6
Standard Costs Using RCC Methodology

	Nursing	Lab	X-ray	P.T.	O.R.
Procedure 1	$240.86588	$37.48883	$34.88722	$55.54549	$15.67138
Procedure 2	$289.03905	$51.54714	$165.71430	$77.76369	$15.67138
Procedure 3	$385.38541	$112.46650	$130.82708	$88.87279	$15.67138

Note: the $240.86588 figure for Procedure 1 for nursing is calculated by multiplying the charge for procedure 1 ($500 from Table 2) by the calculated ratio of costs to charges (.481731757).

She looked at the table. "As I said, the methodology is simple, but not very accurate. RCC might work if prices were based on costs in the first place, but to use it for hospitals that don't have cost accounting systems, and therefore have never known their true costs, is risky," Natalie said.

"They aren't very close to the standard costs we calculated using the RVU methodology," Dr. Amos said.

"The scary thing is, many hospitals are using RCC standard costs in bidding fixed-price contracts," said Natalie.

"Did we use RCC on our Mountainlands bid?" Wes asked.

"We did," replied Natalie.

"From now on, let's use this new methodology."

Supplement Twelve

The Use of Case Mix in Assessing Efficiency

"Did you see the ads our competitor has been running in the paper for the past three days?" Wes asked as the session continued. Removing an ad he clipped from the local newspaper, he handed it to Natalie. "Snowline Regional Medical Center is using this data to claim that they're the most efficient hospital in the valley," he reported. "Their whole advertising campaign is based on their costs, which they say are lower than ours."

"How do they come to that conclusion?" Natalie asked. "I've seen copies of their charges, and they aren't less than ours."

"They used three methodologies," said Wes. In the first ad, they used the same methodology the local grocery stores use in their ads. They picked a dozen or so procedures, totaled the prices of this "shopping basket," then compared the total to ours."

"Who selected the items in the shopping basket?" Natalie asked.

"They did."

"That's part of the problem," she replied. "One can select only those procedures that are priced less, ignoring all others."

They also compared our per-diem rate for medical, surgical, and obstetrics."

"How did they define per-diem?" she asked.

"Is there more than one option?" Wes asked.

"You could price per-diem using billed charges, billed charges less 15 percent, average charges, negotiated charges, or actual reimbursement received. Each will give you a different answer."

"They used billed charges," said Wes.

"That's probably not a fair methodology," said Natalie. "Few patients pay billed charges."

"In the second ad, they compare our basic room rates for medical, surgical, pediatric, and obstetrics nursing units," continued Wes.

"Yeah, but they play games with their rate schedules," said Natalie. "Most patients focus on the daily room rate when comparing hospital prices; what they fail to understand, however, is that 60 to 70 percent of a total hospital bill is ancillary charges. Their ancillary charges are dramatically higher than ours."

"Isn't it also true their average lenght-of-stay is longer?" asked Wes.

"That's right. Our basic room rate for a medical admission is $200 a day. Theirs is $180. Our average lenght-of-stay is three days, however, which gives us a room charge per admission of $600. Their average lenght-of-stay is 4.5 days, which makes their average room charge $810."

"What about their third ad?" asked Wes. "In this one they take the average actual cost from four diagnostic categories. The data comes from the Medicare database, which should be accurate. Don't those data show they are more cost efficient than we are?"

"Not necessarily," said Natalie. "It depends on the case mix of each hospital compared."

"You may have told me before, but what is *case mix*?" asked Wes.

"Case mix refers to the acuity or intensity of illness of the average patient admitted to a specific hospital. Medicare computes a case mix index for all hospitals, based on the mix of diagnoses they treat. Specialty hospitals like the University Hospital, that treat more severe illnesses, have a higher case mix index than community hospitals that refer those critically ill patients elsewhere. It only makes sense that a specialty hospital would have a higher average cost than a community hospital. While our case mix index is not as high as that of the University Hospital, I know it's higher than that of Snowline Regional Medical Center."

"Can you show me how case mix is calculated?" asked Wes.

"I think so," said Natalie. "Again, I'll use my laptop computer and project the data on the screen so that all of you can see it." The group took a five minute break while Natalie created her data set. When they reconvened, she began.

"Let's assume, for the sake of simplifying this model that there are only three hospitals in the world," said Natalie, "Peter Brannan Community Hospital, Snowline Regional Medical Center and University Hospital. Let's also assume that there are only four DRGs."

"That should simplify things," said Wes.

"When the DRG system first came out, Medicare determined the average cost of each DRG through the Medicare Cost Report hospitals submit each year."

"I though you said hospitals didn't know product costs," Wes said.

"They used charges as a *surrogate* for costs," said Natalie. "It wasn't as accurate, but that was all they had. Let's assume they determined the following data on the only three hospitals in our model world." Natalie projected the data on the screen.

Table 1
Actual Revenue for 1995 by DRG for Peter Brannan Community Hospital

1	2	3	4
	Average Charge	Number of DRGs	Revenue
DRG 1	$6,200	520	$3,224,000
DRG 2	$3,140	610	$1,915,400
DRG 3	$4,600	400	$1,840,000
DRG 4	$5,250	400	$2,100,000
Total		1,930	$9,079,400
Average			$4,704

Column Definitions:

Column 1: The diagnostic related group.
Column 2: The actual revenue collected for each DRG, divided by the actual number of DRGs. Revenue includes payment by many individuals and insurance companies under multiple payment systems.
Column 3: The actual number of patients seen whose disease places them in the specific DRG.

Column 4: The actual revenue collected for each DRG. Revenue includes payment by many individuals and insurance companies under multiple payment systems.

Table 2
Actual Revenue for 1995 by DRG for Snowline Regional Medical Center

	Average Charge	Number of DRGs	Revenue
DRG 1	$6,110	250	$1,527,500
DRG 2	$2,860	300	$858,000
DRG 3	$5,510	110	$606,100
DRG 4	$5,950	50	$297,500
Total		710	$3,289,100
Average			$4,633

Table 3
Actual Revenue for 1995 by DRG for University Hospital

	Average Charge	Number of DRGs	Revenue
DRG 1	$7,010	75	$525,750
DRG 2	$3,390	20	$67,800
DRG 3	$8,240	220	$1,812,800
DRG 4	$5,590	60	$335,400
Total Revenue		375	$2,741,750
Average Charge			$7,311

"I have given you the same data for all hospitals: average billed charge per DRG, the total number of DRGs billed, and total revenue. Notice I have also calculated an average charge for each hospital. That's essentially what Snowline published in its ad. A figure calculated by taking total revenues and dividing by total procedures."

"That's not a meaningful figure to use for cost comparison," said Wes. "Those hospitals with a greater percentage of expensive DRGs would have higher average costs."

"That's correct," said Natalie. "The mix of cases seen by a hospital makes a difference. That's why it's important to know something about each hospital's case mix. When Medicare adopted the DRG reimbursement system, it recognized this and developed a methodology to calculate a *case mix index* for each hospital. Let me show you how that's done," she said, as she focused again on her computer.

"Lets go back to our model world—the one with three hospitals and four DRGs. After Medicare collected the data shown in Tables 1, 2, and 3, it calculated the average charge nationally for each DRG. For our model, this calculation is shown in Table 4."

Table 4

Calculation of Average Charge for Each DRG Based on Three Hospitals' Data

	Total Charges	Number of DRGs	Average Charge	Case Mix Index for DRG
DRG 1	$5,227,250	845	$6,245	1.0000
DRG 2	$2,841,200	930	$3,055	.4892
DRG 3	$4,258,900	730	$5,834	.9342
DRG 4	$2,732,900	510	$5,359	.8580

Notes on table calculations:

- To determine average charge, divide total charges by number of DRGs.
- To determine Case Mix Index for DRG, divide each average charge by the highest average charge. For DRG 2, the calculation is $3,055/$6,245 = .4892.

"To calculate a case mix index, take one of the average charges and divide all other charges by that figure. In this case, I used DRG 1 as the base figure. Divide $6,245 by $6,245, and you get 1.000. Divide $3,055 by $6,245, and you get .4892."

"I now understand how case mix indexes are calculated for DRGs," said Wes. "A case mix index is like the RVUs we discussed at the retreat."

"Right, case mix indexes are relative value units," said Natalie. "They measure the relative cost of different DRGs. After Medicare calculated the case mix index for each DRG, it was easy to calculate a hospital's case mix index. Let me demonstrate that methodology for the three model hospitals in Tables 5, 6 and 7."

Table 5

Calculation of Case mix Index—Peter Brannan Community Hospital

1	2	3	4
Diagnostic Related Group	Case Mix Index	Number	Total
DRG 1	1.0000	520	520.0000
DRG 2	.4892	610	298.3992
DRG 3	.9342	400	373.6660
DRG 4	.8580	400	343.2121
Total		1,930	1535.274
Case mix index			.7955

Definitions of Column Headings:

Column 1: The specific DRG.
Column 2: The case mix index calculated by Medicaid using data from all acute care hospitals in the United States.
Column 3: The number of each cases sees during the period by Peter Brannan Community Hospital.
Column 4: The number shown in column 2 times the number shown in column 3. The original calculation done in Excel used numbers with more decimal places than that displayed, hence the rounding errors for the last four digits of the figures shown in column 4.

"The case mix index for Peter Brannan Community Hospital is calculated by multiplying the case mix index by the number of individual DRGs performed during the year. The case mix index is determined by dividing that total figure—1535.2774 in this example—by the total DRGs performed, which is 1,930 in this instance. For this model of Peter Brannan Community Hospital, the case mix index is .7955."

"What does that mean?" asked Wes.

"It means that the severity of the illnesses of our patients, as evidenced by our mix of patients, indicates that we spend 79.55 percent as much money treating our average patient as a hospital that had a case mix index of 1.0000. Let me finish the calculations to explain how this works. Let's calculate the case mix index for Snowline and University Hospitals.

Table 6
Calculation of Case mix Index—Snowline Regional Medical Center

	Case Mix Index	Number	Total
DRG 1	1.0000	250	250.0000
DRG 2	.4892	300	146.7537
DRG 3	.9342	110	102.7582
DRG 4	.8580	50	42.9015
Total		710	542.4134
Case mix index			.7640

Table 7
Calculation of Case mix Index—University Hospital

	Case Mix Index	Number	Total
DRG 1	1.0000	75	75.0000
DRG 2	.4892	20	9.7836
DRG 3	.9342	220	205.5163
DRG 4	.8580	60	51.4818
Total		375	341.7817
Case mix index			.9114

"You will notice from the data that each hospital has a different case mix index. The hospital with the highest case mix index is University Hospital, with an index of .9114. Snowline has the lowest case mix index. We are in between."

"This is all fine and well, but how does it help me determine which hospital is most cost efficient?" asked Wes.

"The best way to compare hospitals on the basis of cost efficiency is to divide the hospital's *average charge* by its *case mix index*. This provides a *case mix adjusted average charge* that can be more accurately used in comparing the true costs of competing hospitals. Let's do that calculation," she said. "The calculation is made by dividing the average charge calculated in Tables 1, 2 and 3 by the case mixes of the individual hospitals. It works like this."

Table 8
Calculation of Case Mix Adjusted Charges for Three Hospitals

	Peter Brannan Community Hospital	Snowline Regional Medical Center	University Hospital
Average charge	$4,704	$4,633	$7,311
Case mix index	.7955	.7640	.9114
Case mix adjusted average charge	$5,914	$6,064	$8,022

"From these data, you can see that the newspaper ad was wrong. Snowline Regional Medical Center may have the lowest average charge, but without a case-mix adjustment, this figure is meaningless, as we discussed earlier. When we make that adjustment, Peter Brannan Community Hospital has the lowest adjusted charge. This is the best surrogate for cost efficiency we have."

"Let's do the full set of calculations and get this information to the newspaper," Wes said.

"It's done," said Natalie.

Supplement Thirteen

Rolling up Standard Procedure Costs to Determine Product Costs

Later that day, Wes Douglas and his team gathered again in the living room of Dr. Amos's cabin. Wes began the discussion. "We need," he paused, "to determine final product costs. For our first model, let's define two types of final products—DRGs and Capitation Payment enrollees. Now that we have standard costs per procedure, we can roll these up into standard costs for individual products."

"This is a fairly easy calculation," said Natalie. "Let me model it on my computer. I'll project the data on the screen."

Natalie was silent for a few minutes while she entered data for the model. When the model was finished, she spoke. "For simplicity in building our model, let's assume only four DRGs. Table 1 lists the fixed payment the model hospital receives from the government for each DRG and the number of DRGs it performs each year. Also, included at the bottom is the yearly amount received from one insurance company that pays on a capitation payment basis. The company pays $540 per year per enrollee in its HMO.

Table 1
DRG Data—Model Hospital

Billing System	Payment	Number Provided
DRG 1	$5,800	500
DRG 2	$2,500	500
DRG 3	$3,800	400
DRG 4	$4,500	400
Yearly Capitation Pmt	$1,500	1,500

"Let's start with DRG 1. Our first step is to examine medical records and determine the average cost of procedures provided to a patient in this DRG classification. Let's assume the study determined the following:

Table 2
Resources Used in Treating DRG 1

1	2	1	2
Resource	Number	Resource	Number
Nursing:		Physical Therapy"	
Procedure 1	4	Procedure 1	3
Procedure 2	2	Procedure 2	1
Procedure 3	2	Procedure 3	0
Lab:		Operating Room:	
Procedure 1	6	Procedure 1	90
Procedure 2	2	Procedure 2	0
Procedure 3	3	Procedure 3	0
X-ray:			
Procedure 1	1		
Procedure 2	4		
Procedure 3	4		

Definition of column headings:

Column 1: The names of the procedures used to treat DRG 1.
Column 2: The number of procedures used.

"To determine a final product cost, we would simply sum the costs of each of its component products and procedures, as shown on Table 3."

Table 3
Standard Cost for DRG 1

1	2	3	4
Resource	#	Standard Cost	Total Standard Cost
Nursing			
Procedure 1	4	$136.92	$547.69
Procedure 2	2	$393.77	$787.54
Procedure 3	2	$591.69	$1,183.39
Lab			
Procedure 1	6	$47.61	$285.66
Procedure 2	2	$33.81	$67.61
Procedure 3	3	$105.42	$316.25
X-ray			
Procedure 1	1	$57.61	$57.61
Procedure 2	4	$148.02	$592.07
Procedure 3	4	$123.41	$493.64
Phys Therapy			
Procedure 1	3	$56.63	$169.89
Procedure 2	1	$72.17	$72.17
Procedure 3	0	$96.72	$0.00
Operating Room			
Procedure 1	90	$8.41	$756.48
Procedure 2	0	$14.81	$0
Procedure 3	0	$23.22	$0
Total DRG Cost			**$5,330**

Definition of Column Headings:

Column 1: The names of the procedures used to treat DRG 1.
Column 2: The number of procedures used.
Column 3: The standard cost of the individual procedure, as determined by the methodology explained earlier in the textbook.
Column 4: The product of column 3 times column 4.

"In this example, we are paid $5,800 for DRG 1 (see table 1). Our standard costs are $5,330. We make, therefore, $470 on average on each case, provided actual cost parallels standard cost."

Cost Roll ups for Capitation Payment

"That sounds simple enough," Wes said. "But what do we do to roll up costs for comparison to capitation payment reimbursement?"

"We use a different methodology." She wrote the following steps to the calculation on the board:

1. *Sort all enrollees into demographic categories by age and sex.*
2. *Have an actuary determine the number of hospital admissions we can expect by demographic category.*

3. *Have an actuary determine the diseases these patients will have.*
4. *Use the resource profile, to determine what procedures we will have to provide for each patient.*
5. *Multiply the number of procedures by their total standard costs.*
6. *Calculate total costs by demographic category.*
7. *Divide total costs by demographic category by the number of enrollee months to determine the cost per enrollee per month*
8. *Compare the cost per enrollee per month with the capitation payment we will receive.*

At the conclusion of this discussion, the group took a fifteen minute break.

Calculating Product Cost Variances before and after the Installation of the Complete Cost Accounting System

When the group reconvened, Natalie was the first to speak. "What we are describing is a fairly complex process. To keep from getting lost in the detail, let's return for a moment to our original objective, the calculation of cost variances. Does anyone remember how variances are calculated?" she asked.

"It is the difference between standard cost per procedure, and actual cost per procedure," said Wes.

"That's correct," she said. "All we have done so far is to demonstrate a methodology to calculate standard cost per procedure. Capturing actual cost per procedure is more difficult for hospitals than it is for manufacturing companies."

"Why is that?" Elizabeth asked.

"Because hospitals have so many products—30,000 at some hospitals—that are not uniform, patient to patient."

"What do you mean by that?" Elizabeth asked.

"Is the time it requires to give a shot to a healthy 40 year old female the same as the time it requires to give the same shot to a terrorized three year old?"

"Probably not."

"We can't assume the same uniformity of products, that we have in process costing. And we don't have the technology to collect accurate actual cost data using job costing because of the number of products we offer."

"What are you trying to tell us?" Wes asked.

"If you are manufacturing computer boards using a process costing system it is possible to accurately capture the labor and materials actually used per batch. Dividing batch costs by the number of units in the batch will give a per-unit cost. We can't batch patients, however, as the resources used to deliver a basic procedure vary from patient to patient, depending upon his or her age, severity of illness, and whether or not he or she is conscious, bedridden, etc.

"If you are building custom homes using job order costing, it is possible to accurately capture the actual labor and materials by home. You can't do that in a hospital, there are too many products and procedures. It isn't cost effective to record the time that every procedure takes to deliver to every patient. Hospitals, as a rule, don't capture actual labor costs by patient. Consequently, their ability to calculate accurate labor variances is limited."

"Until the technology is there to capture the data in a cost effective manner, is there any type of variance analysis that we can perform?" Elizabeth asked.

"We can't calculate variances on a per-product or per-procedure basis," Natalie said. "But we can calculate them at the department level. The data isn't as useful, but, gives some information."

"Show us what department level variances look like," Wes said.

For the next few minutes, Natalie prepared an illustration of department level variances, shown below:

Table 4
Variance Analysis for July 1995
Laboratory Department—Model Hospital

	Procedure 1	Procedure 2	Procedure 3	Total
Number of procedures performed	1,200	550	200	1,950
Standard direct labor dollars per procedure	$24	$12	$36	
Standard direct labor dollars	$28,800	$6,600	$7,200	$42,600
Actual direct labor from payroll ledger				$47,500
Total variance direct labor dollars				($4,900)
Standard direct material per procedure	$12	$16	$52	
Standard direct materials	$14,400	$8,800	$10,400	$33,600
Actual direct materials				$37,100
Total variance direct materials				($3,500)
Standard fixed department overhead				$20,833
Actual fixed department overhead				$20,000
Total variance fixed department overhead				$833

Note: Although not shown above, a variable overhead variance could also be produced, if there is variable overhead.

"With standard costs per procedure and actual costs per department, all we can produce are three total variances: a direct labor variance, a direct materials variance, and a fixed overhead variance," said Natalie. "And knowing the variances doesn't tell us what caused them. If there is a labor variance, for example, we don't know if it is a rate or a efficiency variance."

"The information isn't as useful as more detailed variances would be," said Elizabeth, "but until the technology exists to capture actual cost by procedure, it is better than nothing."

✳ ✳ ✳

At the conclusion of the retreat, Natalie Simpson prepared a summary of the model, which is found on the next page. This is a good review for hospital accountants who are interested in installing a cost accounting system at their own hospital.

Cost Accounting Model

This is a model that can be used as a review of the principles taught in this book, or as a tool in training new accounting personnel on the basics of hospital cost accounting.   To download an Excel copy, go to the author's web page: http://www.traemus-books.com

Supplement 14

Standard Cost Accounting System Illustrated

In building a standard cost model, the first thing we need to do is determine the standard cost for each primary product or service. Standard cost per product consists of standard direct labor, standard direct materials, and standard overhead. We will use an RVU-based methodology to determine standard cost. Other options discussed in the text include conducting an industrial engineered study, borrowing standards from professional organizations or other hospitals, etc.

To simplify the model, let's assume our hospital has only three revenue producing *departments: Nursing, Laboratory, and Pharmacy. To simplify terminology, we will refer to all products and all services as "products."*

First, we determine what the primary products are in each revenue department. In our example, the primary products in nursing are called *patient days*. The primary products in laboratory are called *laboratory tests*, and the primary products in pharmacy are *prescriptions*.

Our next step is to determine how many labor RVUs it takes to complete a product. Remember, a laboratory test with an RVU of 2 takes twice as much labor as a test with an RVU of 1. It is the *relative* weights that are important with RVUs. We will assume in this case that we obtained RVU data from professional organizations. These are summarized in Table 1.

In Table 1, we also show the variable material per product. The easiest way to get this information is to pull invoices.

Table 1— Relative Value Units (RVUs) value and Variable Material per Revenue Department

Product	Nursing			Laboratory			Pharmacy		
	Acuity 1	Acuity 2	Acuity 3	Lab Test A	Lab Test B	Lab Test C	Rx 1	Rx 2	Rx 3
RVU/ Unit	1	2.5	3.7	1	4	7	1	1.5	3
Variable Material	$30.00	$60.00	$80.00	$4.00	$9.00	$15.00	$1.00	$1.50	$3.00

The next table pulls RVU information and payroll information into one table. See the definitions at the bottom of the table to understand where the numbers shown in each column come from.

Table 2—RVUs and Department Payroll by Month

1	2	3	4	5	6	7
Month	Total RVUs Nursing	Total Labor Costs Nursing	Total RVUs Laboratory	Total Labor Costs Laboratory	Total RVUs Pharmacy	Total Labor Costs Pharmacy
Jan	2,318	$ 127,900.00	13,010	$ 154,755.38	225	$ 1,225.00
Feb	2,297	$ 126,850.00	13,430	$ 158,854.58	193	$ 1,193.00
Mar	2,224	$ 123,200.00	13,100	$ 155,633.78	258	$ 1,258.00
Apr	2,534	$ 138,700.00	13,670	$ 161,196.98	262	$ 1,262.00
May	2,266	$ 125,300.00	13,070	$ 155,340.98	164	$ 1,164.00
Jun	2,227	$ 123,350.00	12,990	$ 154,560.18	222	$ 1,222.00
Jul	2,420	$ 133,000.00	13,750	$ 161,977.78	259	$ 1,259.00
Aug	2,600	$ 142,000.00	12,900	$ 153,681.78	181	$ 1,181.00
Sep	2,479	$ 135,950.00	12,640	$ 151,144.18	314	$ 1,314.00
Oct	2,166	$ 120,300.00	12,220	$ 147,044.98	321	$ 1,321.00
Nov	2,323	$ 128,150.00	12,540	$ 150,168.18	353	$ 1,353.00
Dec	2,497	$ 136,850.00	13,220	$ 156,804.98	292	$ 1,292.00
Total	28,351	$ 1,561,550.00	156,540	$ 1,861,163.73	3,044	$ 15,044.00

Definitions of Data Found in Each Column:

Column 1: The month for which the data was collected.

Column 2: The total number of relative value units for the month. This could be calculated by multiplying the number of each product produced in the department by its relative value unit. For example, if we produced 1,000 units of product 1 during the month, and each product 1 had an RVU of 5, the total RVUs for product 1 would be 5,000. If there were three products in the department, we would add the total RVUs from each of the three products to get the amount shown in Column 2. In this example you haven't been given the number of products in each department, we calculated the total RVUs for you. In this example, the number shown in Column 2 is given.

Column 3: This is the total labor cost for the department, taken from payroll records.

Column 4: Same as definition for Column 2, except the data is for Laboratory.

Column 5: Same as definition as for Column 3, except the data is for Laboratory.

234

Column 6: Same as definition for Column 2, except the data is for Pharmacy.
Column 7: Same as the definition for Column 3, except the data is for Pharmacy.

Using the RVUs and labor cost information, we separate variable labor costs into fixed and variable components for each revenue department. To do this we use the Least Squares Method (i.e. multiple regression) as demonstrated in the textbook/novel. In this example, I used the regression program from Excel. The relevant portion of the output from Excel is as follows:

Table 3—Regression Output

Regression Statistics						
Multiple R	1					
R Square	1					
Adjusted R Square	1					
Standard Error	1.1822E-10					
Observations	11					
	Coefficients	Standard Error	t Stat	P-value	Lower 95%	Upper 95%
Intercept	12000	6.08817E-10	1.97104E+13	1.134E-116	12000	12000
X Coefficient	50	2.56809E-13	1.94697E+14	1.2666E-125	50	50

The R Square shows how well the model works. An R Square of 1.00 means x and y have a perfect relationship. The reason our R Square is 1.00 is that we made the data up to illustrate the technique. Usually you won't get a perfect R square. The intercept shown on the table is 12,000. That means that our monthly fixed costs are $12,000. The X Coefficient is 50. That tells us our variable cost is $50 per relative value unit (not variable cost per product but relative cost per RVU—remember we regressed on relative value units).

Using the data from the excel output, we put this data into a cost formula. The three formulas for our three departments are:

General formula: $Y = a + bx$; or $Y =$ fixed costs + (variable cost per RVU x number of RVUs)

Nursing: $y = \$12,000 + \$50.00x$

Laboratory: $y = \$27,777.78 + \$9.76x$

Pharmacy: $y = \$1,000 + \$1.00x$

Now, let's take the variable labor cost per RVU and convert it into variable labor cost per primary product; patient day for Nursing, lab test for Laboratory, and prescription (Rx) for Pharmacy.

Table 4 — Standard Cost Table – Labor

		Nursing			Laboratory			Pharmacy		
1										
2	Product	Acuity 1	Acuity 2	Acuity 3	Lab Test A	Lab Test B	Lab Test C	Rx 1	Rx 2	Rx 3
3	Variable labor cost per RVU	$50.00	$50.00	$50.00	$9.76	$9.76	$9.76	$1.00	$1.00	$1.00
4	RVU per product	1	2.5	3.7	1	4	7	1	2	3
5	Variable Labor cost per product	$50.00	$125.00	$185.00	$9.76	$39.04	$68.32	$1.00	$2.00	$3.00

Definition of Data Found in Each Row:

Row 1: The name of each of the three departments in our model hospital.
Row 2: The name of each individual product in each of the three departments. In the model, each department has three products.
Row 3: The variable labor per RVU, as determined using the least squared methodology above.
Row 4: The labor RVUs per product, given earlier.
Row 5: The answer we receive when we multiply the number in Row 4 by the number in Row 5. This is the variable labor cost per product.

Now that we have calculated the variable labor for each product, we add this figure to the variable materials for each product to give us total variable costs for each product. In our example, we assume that all overhead was fixed—that there was no variable overhead. If there were variable overhead, then that would be added in as well to give us the total variable costs shown in Row 5.

Table 5—Standard Cost Table – Variable Costs

1		Nursing			Laboratory			Pharmacy		
2	Product	Acuity 1	Acuity 2	Acuity 3	Lab Test A	Lab Test B	Lab Test C	Rx 1	Rx 2	Rx 3
3	Variable Labor per Product	$50.00	$125.00	$185.00	$9.76	$39.04	$68.32	$1.00	$1.50	$3.00
4	Variable Materials per Product	$30.00	$60.00	$80.00	$4.00	$9.00	$15.00	$1.00	$1.50	$3.00
5	Total Variable per Product	$80.00	$185.00	$265.00	$13.76	$48.04	$83.32	$2.00	$3.00	$6.00

The figures in Row 5 are calculated by summing the figures in Row 3 and Row 4.

Now, look at the data. Notice we have calculated total variable costs per patient day in Nursing, per lab test in Laboratory, and per prescription in the Pharmacy.

By creating a subtotal for variable costs, we facilitate cost-volume-profit analysis and break-even analysis, etc.

Next, we need to allocate department overhead costs to each patient day, lab test, or prescription. The fixed overhead material costs are found in the general ledger. The fixed overhead labor costs come from the regressions we ran earlier. Since these fixed costs were per month, we multiply by twelve to get the annual fixed labor costs. Other fixed costs would include supplies, depreciation, utility bills, etc. The total number of primary products (patient days, lab tests, or prescriptions) are found in department records.

Table 6—Standard Cost Table—Department Overhead

		Nursing	Laboratory	Pharmacy
1				
2	Fixed Labor Costs	$ 144,000.00	$ 333,333.33	$ 12,000.00
3	Fixed Materials Costs	96,000.00	80,000.00	15,000.00
4	Other Expense	120,000.00	150,000.00	70,000.00
5	Total Department Overhead	$ 360,000.00	$ 563,333.33	$ 97,000.00
6				
7	Calculation Of Department Overhead Rate: (Total Department Overhead/Units of Primary Product)			
8				
9	Total Primary Products			
10	Patient Days	11,020.00		
11	Lab Tests		33,630	
12	Rxs			2,328
13				
14	Rate Per Primary Product	$ 32.6679	$ 16.7509	$ 41.6666

Notes on Calculations:

Row 2 is calculated by multiplying the monthly fixed costs calculated earlier using Least Squares by 12 (the number of months in a year)

Row 3 is taken from purchasing records.

Row 4 is taken from the general ledger. It is given in this example.

Row 10, 11 and 12 are taken from department records.

Row 14 is the rate used in allocating fixed overhead to products. It is calculated by dividing the amount summed in row 5, by either the figure shown in row 10 (for nursing), or Row 11 (for lab), or Row 12 (for pharmacy).

Now we have more information to add to our standard cost table.

Table 7—Standard Cost Table – Variable Costs

Primary Product	Nursing			Laboratory			Pharmacy		
	Acuity 1	Acuity 2	Acuity3	Lab Test A	Lab Test B	Lab Test C	Rx 1	Rx 2	Rx 3
Variable Labor per Product	$50.00	$125.00	$185.00	$9.76	$39.04	$68.32	$1.00	$1.50	$3.00
Variable Materials per Product	$30.00	$60.00	$80.00	$4.00	$9.00	$15.00	$1.00	$1.50	$3.00
Total Variable per Product	$80.00	$185.00	$265.00	$13.76	$48.04	$83.32	$2.00	$3.00	$6.00
Dept. OH per Product*	$32.67	$32.67	$32.67	$16.75	$16.75	$16.75	$41.67	$41.67	$41.67
Total Cost per Product	$112.67	$217.67	$297.67	$30.51	$64.79	$100.07	$43.67	$44.67	$47.67

* Rounded to two decimals (throughout)

Thus far, we have assigned direct labor, direct materials, and department overhead to our primary products. We will now assign General Hospital Overhead. This includes the costs of all non-revenue producing departments (service departments) such as Finance, Laundry, and Housekeeping. For our example, these costs are given as $400,000 for Finance, $190,000 for Laundry, and $230,000 for Housekeeping.

In this example, we will allocate these costs using the double apportionment method (you could also use the direct method, step method, or reciprocal method). We will allocate general hospital overhead using number of financial transactions as the allocation base for the Finance Department, pounds of laundry as the allocation base for the Laundry, and department square feet as the allocation base for Housekeeping.

Remember, this is the double apportionment method, demonstrated earlier in the textbook. Let's show the calculation of rates for the first apportionment.

Table 8—Overhead Allocation – Step 1

	Finance	Laundry	Housekeeping	Nursing	Lab	Pharmacy	Base
Allocation Statistics							
Number of financial transactions			980	3480	2100	4890	12,500
Pounds of laundry	400		5000	24000	8000	2000	39,400
Square feet	3500	5600		29000	5000	6500	49,600
Service Department Costs	$ 400,000.00	$ 190,000.00	$ 230,000.00				
Allocate Finance	$ (400,000.00)	33,600.00	31,360.00	111,360.00	67,200.00	156,480.00	
Allocate Laundry	2,270.05	$ (223,600.00)	28,375.63	136,203.05	45,401.02	11,350.25	
Allocate Housekeeping	$ 20,445.05	$ 32,712.09	$ (289,735.63)	$ 169,401.88	$ 29,207.22	$ 37,969.39	
Balance after first allocation	$ 22,715.11	$ 32,712.09	$ -	$ 416,964.93	$ 141,808.24	$ 205,799.64	

Some explanation may be useful. The data in the "Allocation Statistics" is obtained from records kept by the individual service departments. We wish to allocate service department costs to the three revenue producing departments. With double apportionment, the first step is to allocate each service department to *all* other departments, service and revenue. For Finance, our rate is $32.00 ($400,000/12,500) per financial transactions. Laundry's rate is $5.67 ($223,600/39,400) per pound of laundry, and Housekeeping's base allocated at $5.84 ($289,735.63/49,600) per square foot.

We will allocate what is left in the service departments after the first allocation using a step-down methodology. We need to calculate new rates. This time, we will not allocate to previous departments. The allocation base will include only the allocation statistics from departments to the right of the department being allocated. The allocation bases, therefore, are Number of financial transactions = 12,500; Pounds of laundry = 39,000; Square feet = 40,500.

240

Table 9—Overhead Allocation – Step 2

	Finance	Laundry	Housekeeping	Nursing	Lab	Pharmacy	Base
Allocation Statistics							
Number of financial transactions		1050	980	3480	2100	4890	12,500
Pounds of laundry			5000	24000	8000	2000	39,000
Square feet				29000	5000	6500	40,500
Service Department Costs	$ 22,715.11	$ 32,712.09					
Allocate Finance	$ (22,715.11)	1,908.07	1,780.86	6,323.89	3,816.14	8,886.15	
Allocate Laundry		$ (34,620.16)	4,438.48	21,304.71	7,101.57	1,775.39	
Allocate Housekeeping			$ (6,219.35)	$ 4,453.36	$ 767.82	$ 998.17	
Balance after 2nd allocation				$ 32,081.96	$ 11,685.53	$ 11,659.71	

Next, we total the sum of overhead allocated from the two allocation steps to get the total allocation from service departments to revenue departments.

Table 10—Total Allocation

	Nursing	Laboratory	Pharmacy	Total
First allocation	$ 416,964.93	$ 141,808.24	$ 205,799.64	$ 764,572.81
Second allocation	$ 32,081.96	$ 11,685.53	$ 11,659.71	$ 55,427.19
Total allocation	$ 449,046.88	$ 153,493.77	$ 217,459.35	$ 820,000.00

We now have the allocation of general hospital costs to the revenue departments. Let's refine this to an allocation per primary product within each revenue department.

Table 11—Calculation of General Hospital Overhead Rate Per Product

	Nursing	Lab	Pharmacy
Allocated Overhead	$ 449,046.88	$ 153,493.77	$ 217,459.35
Patient Days	11,020		
Lab Tests		33,630	
Prescriptions (Rx)			2,328
Overhead rate per Product	$ 40.7484	$ 4.5642	$ 93.4104

Now we have the information we need to complete the standard cost for the revenue departments.

Table 12—Standard Cost Table – Complete

Product	Nursing			Laboratory			Pharmacy		
	Acuity 1	Acuity 2	Acuity3	Lab Test A	Lab Test B	Lab Test C	Rx 1	Rx 2	Rx 3
Variable Labor per Primary Product	$50.00	$125.00	$185.00	$9.76	$39.04	$68.32	$1.00	$1.50	$3.00
Variable Materials per Primary Product	$30.00	$60.00	$80.00	$4.00	$9.00	$15.00	$1.00	$1.50	$3.00
Total Variable Costs per Primary Product	$80.00	$185.00	$265.00	$13.76	$48.04	$83.32	$2.00	$3.00	$6.00
Department Overhead per Primary Product	$32.67	$32.67	$32.67	$16.75	$16.75	$16.75	$41.67	$41.67	$41.67
Department Cost per Primary Product	$112.67	$217.67	$297.67	$30.51	$64.79	$100.07	$43.67	$44.67	$47.67
Allocated Hospital Overhead per Primary Product	$40.75	$40.75	$40.75	$4.56	$4.56	$4.56	$93.41	$93.41	$93.41
Total Standard Cost per Product	$153.42	$258.42	$338.42	$35.07	$69.35	$104.63	$137.08	$138.08	$141.08

243

As mentioned in the text, our hospital rolls the costs of primary products into secondary products, and rolls the cost of secondary products into final products. To simplify the illustration, however, in this example we are going to assume only two levels of products, primary and final. Table 12 shows the cost per primary product. Now let's roll our costs up into a final product, DRG 777. Assume our product consumption profile shows that the average patient classified into DRG 777 consumes 3 Acuity Level 1 patient days, one Acuity Level 3 patient days, one lab test A, two lab test Bs, and five test Cs, 3 Rx 1s, 2 Rx 2s, and 5 Rx 3s. What would be the standard cost for DRG 777? Let's roll it up and see!

Management Report 1
Standard Cost for Final Product DRG 777

Primary Product	Standard Cost of One Primary Product	Number of Primary Products Consumed	Total Cost
Acuity 1 patient day	$ 153.4162	3	$ 460.25
Acuity 3 patient day	338.4162	1	338.42
Lab test A	35.0751	1	35.08
Lab Test B	69.3551	2	138.71
Lab Test C	104.6351	5	523.18
Rx 1	137.0770	3	411.23
Rx 2	138.0770	2	276.15
Rx 3	141.0770	5	705.39
Total standard Cost for DRG 777			$ 2,888.40

Let's assume our hospital treats patients in only seven DRG categories, and that standard costs are used as a surrogate for actual costs. Which DRGs are profitable to the hospital, and which are not?

Management Report 2
Profitability of Individual DRGs

	DRG Reimbursement	DRG Standard Cost	Profit (Loss)
DRG 2	$ 2,590.00	$ 3,102.00	$ (512.00)
DRG 34	$ 12,557.00	$ 10,995.00	$ 1,562.00
DRG 56	$ 3,402.00	$ 2,001.00	$ 1,401.00
DRG 132	$ 5,463.00	$ 6,690.00	$ (1,227.00)
DRG 226	$ 1,200.00	$ 1,450.00	$ (250.00)
DRG 358	$ 7,080.00	$ 9,000.00	$ (1,920.00)
DRG 777	$ 3,200.90	$ 2,888.40	$ 312.50

<u>Definition of Data Found in Each Column:</u>

Column 1: Name of DRG.
Column 2: Fixed payment we receive for each DRG. This is determined by Medicare.
Column 3: Standard cost for each DRG as determined using methodology shown above.
Column 4: The difference between payment and cost—the profit or loss.

From this report, we see that every time we perform DRG 358, we are paid $1,920. Every time we perform DRG 34, we will generate a profit of $1,562. Useful information!

Let's produce some additional reports. Assume we are concerned about Dr. Smith who consistently uses more resources than other physicians. We can pull the chart on twenty of his patients and compare his resource profile for DRG 777 to our standards.

245

Management Report 3
Dr. Smith's Cost Profile on DRG 777

DRG 777 Resources	Standard Usage	Dr. Smith's Average Usage	Usage Variance in Units	Standard Cost per Unit	Usage Variance in Dollars
Acuity 1 patient day	3.00	4.2	(1.20)	$ 153.42	$ (184.10)
Acuity 3 patient day	1.00	1.1	(0.10)	$ 338.42	$ (33.84)
Lab Test A	1.00	1	-	$ 35.08	$ -
Lab Test B	2.00	1.5	0.50	$ 69.36	$ 34.68
Lab Test C	5.00	7	(2.00)	$ 104.64	$ (209.27)
Rx 1	3.00	4.5	(1.50)	$ 137.08	$ (205.62)
Rx 2	2.00	4.5	(2.50)	$ 138.08	$ (345.19)
Rx 3	5.00	6.1	(1.10)	$ 141.08	$ (943.34)
Total					$ (1,886.68)

Definition of Data from Each Column:

Column 1: The name of the resource used to treat the patient in DRG 777.
Column 2: The standard quantity.
Column 3: Dr. Smith's actual quantity.
Column 4: The difference between standard and actual for Dr. Smith.
Column 5: The standard cost per primary product as determined using the methodology shown above.
Column 6: The variance for Dr. Smith.

On average, it costs $1888 more for Dr. Smith to treat a patient than the standard. If his outcomes are better, then maybe we should change the standard. If not, Dr. Smith may wish to evaluate his practice pattern.

Now let's prepare a management report on DRG 777 by physician, showing how much we actually make or lose on this diagnosis by physician.

Management Report 4
Profit or Loss by Physician on DRG 777

Doctor	Reimbursement	Actual Standard Cost by Physician	Profit or Loss by Physician
Dr. Smith	$ 3,200.90	$ 4,775.08	$ (1,574.18)
Dr. Adams	$ 3,200.90	$ 2,990.54	$ 210.36
Dr. Jones	$ 3,200.90	$ 2,502.34	$ 698.56
Dr. Doe	$ 3,200.90	$ 4,035.98	$ (835.08)
Dr. Harris	$ 3,200.90	$ 2,400.98	$ 799.92

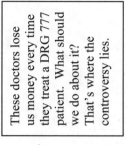

These doctors lose us money every time they treat a DRG 777 patient. What should we do about it? That's where the controversy lies.

Note that we could also calculate the physician's total profitability for the month or year for all DRGs.

Let's now prepare a management report on DRG 777 for the month of December.

Management Report 5
Profit or (Loss) on DRG 777 for Month of December

Patient Number	Patient Age	Length of Stay	Reimbursement if we used Billed Charges	Revenue	Standard Cost	Profit or (Loss)
1002	42	2	$ 3,023.00	$ 3,200.90	$ 2,991.00	$ 209.90
1321	65	3	4,790.00	3,200.90	3,490.00	(289.10)
1356	12	1	1,020.00	3,200.90	2,004.00	1,196.90
1446	34	1	1,209.00	3,200.90	1,440.00	1,760.90
1573	27	1	1,100.00	3,200.90	1,207.00	1,993.90
1695	84	4	6,823.00	3,200.90	5,800.00	(2,599.10)
1708	66	2	3,002.00	3,200.90	2,750.00	450.90
1811	28	2	2,810.00	3,200.90	2,959.00	241.90
1920	48	2	2,689.00	3,200.90	3,105.00	95.90
1999	33	3	4,511.00	3,200.90	4,300.00	(1,099.10)
2109	29	1	1,005.00	3,200.90	1,590.00	1,610.90
			$ 31,982.00	$ 35,209.90	$ 31,636.00	$ 3,573.90

248

What if a new employer approaches us directly and wants to contract with us on a DRG payment basis? We are provided with demographic information on the employees. We give these data to an actuary and receive the following expected utilization for the employee base.

Management Report 6
Expected Profit or Loss for Specific Employer Group

	Expected Utilization	Expected Revenue	Expected Standard Cost	Expected Standard Profit
DRG 2	25	$ 64,750.00	$ 77,550.00	$ (12,800.00)
DRG 34	40	$ 502,280.00	$ 439,800.00	$ 62,480.00
DRG 56	33	$ 112,266.00	$ 66,033.00	$ 46,233.00
DRG 132	12	$ 65,556.00	$ 80,280.00	$ (14,724.00)
DRG 226	17	$ 20,400.00	$ 24,650.00	$ (4,250.00)
DRG 358	53	$ 375,240.00	$ 477,000.00	$ (101,760.00)
DRG 777	19	$ 60,817.10	$ 54,879.60	$ 5,937.50
	199	$ 1,201,309.10	$ 1,220,192.60	$ (18,883.50)

We can expect to lose $18,883.50 a year on this employer. Better find another type of reimbursement, or renegotiate our reimbursement rates.

Definition of Data from Columns:

Column 1: The name of the DRG.
Column 2: The number of cases of the specific DRG that actuaries project the employees in this pool will generate per year.
Column 3: The expected revenue under the billing system we will be using—in this example the figure is given
Column 4: The total standard cost for treating the projected number of cases.
Column 5: The total profit or loss.

Let's assume the above employer comes back to us with a proposal that he/she contract for healthcare services on a capitation payment basis. This employer has 1,000 employees. We want to make 10 percent a year profit on this contract. How much should we charge per month per employee?

Management Report 7
Calculation of Capitation Payment for Specific Employer

Expected standard cost of employee pool*	$ 1,220,192.60
Desired profit of 10%	$ 122,019.26
Desired revenue	$ 1,342,211.86
Number of employee months (1,000 x 12)	12,000
Capitation payment per month	$ 111.85

* See Management Report 6

Rather than examine data by employer or work group, perhaps we want to analyze how much we make by insurance company. Management Report 8 provides us an example of what this might look like. Remember that in all these reports, we assume actual costs are equal to standard costs. If we are more efficient than standard, we would be better off. However, if our actual costs exceed standard, less profit results.

Management Report 8
Profitability by Insurance Company

Insurance Company	Reimbursement Type	Total Reimbursement	Total Standard Costs	Profit or (Loss) by Insurance Co.
Mineral State Ins. Co	Cost reimbursement	$ 403,500.00	$ 302,400.00	$ 101,100.00
Winget Insurance Company	Billed charges	$ 65,899.00	$ 68,009.00	$ (2,110.00)
Green Cross	Capitation	$ 450,667.00	$ 420,987.00	$ 29,680.00
Physicians Mutual	Per Diem	$ 54,390.00	$ 137,000.00	$ (82,610.00)
Medicare	DRG	$ 1,008,960.00	$ 1,000,000.00	$ 8,960.00
Medicaid	DRG	$ 674,000.00	$ 670,000.00	$ 4,000.00
		$ 2,657,416.00	$ 2,598,396.00	$ 59,020.00

With the knowledge of standard costs for each primary product, we can do some flexible budgeting. Assume we project the following activity for Nursing for the year 2002: 3,000 Acuity 1 days, 5,000 Acuity 2 days, and 4,000 Acuity 3 days. What would be the 2000 budget for Nursing?

Management Report 9
Hospital Flexible Budget

Fixed Costs			
Fixed Cost—Labor			$ 144,000.00
Fixed Cost—Materials			$ 96,000.00
Fixed Cost—Other			$ 120,000.00
Total Fixed Costs			$ 360,000.00

Variable Costs	Acuity 1 Pt Days	Acuity 2 Pt Days	Acuity 3 Pt Days	
Variable Labor	$ 50.00	$ 125.00	$ 185.00	
Variable Materials	$ 30.00	$ 60.00	$ 80.00	
Total Variable Department Costs	$ 80.00	$ 185.00	$ 265.00	
Budgeted Days	3,000	5,000	4,000	
Projected variable costs	$ 240,000.00	$ 925,000.00	$ 1,060,000.00	$ 2,225,000.00
Total Department Costs				$ 2,585,000.00

This figure does not include applied General Hospital Overhead.

Let's assume it is now December 31, 2002 and we want to analyze our financial performance for the year. Assume in this situation we had the same number of patient days in each acuity level indicated. What are our variances in Nursing?

252

Management Report 10

	Budget	Actual	Variance
Fixed Costs—Labor	$144,000	$129,000	$15,000
Fixed Costs—Materials	$96,000	$102,000	($6,000)
Fixed Costs—Other	$120,000	$121,000	($1,000)
Variable Labor	$1,515,000	$1,600,111	($85,111)
Variable Materials	$90,000	$88,500	$1,500
Total Dept Cost	$1,965,000	$2,040,611	($75,611)

With our ability to roll up costs, there are many other reports we could produce!

We have an unfavorable total department variance of $75,611. If we wanted to, we could break that into a rate and efficiency variance by obtaining actual payroll hours, labor rates and payroll paid from the Payroll Department. What we cannot do is calculate variances by product, as we currently don't have the technology to track actual cost by product.

Appendix Two

Medical, Economic, and Accounting Terms

Absorption Costing: A type of product costing in which product costs comprise both fixed and variable cost of production. Compare with *Direct Costing.*

Activity Base: The cost driver used in calculating an overhead rate.

Activity Forecasting: The forecasting of the number of goods and services to be provided in a fiscal period.

Actual Cost: Costs actually incurred. Compare with Standard Cost.

Actual Cost Accounting: An accounting system that debits to work-in-process actual direct labor, actual direct materials, and actual overhead. Compare with Standard Cost Accounting.

Actuary: A certified professional specializing in the mathematics of risk and insurance.

Acuity of Illness: A numeric index denoting the complexity of the goods and services needed to treat a diagnosis.

Administrator: See Hospital Administrator.

Admission: The term applied to each person admitted for care to the hospital.

Allocation Base for Service Departments: The unit of output that has been identified for use in allocating service department costs to revenue departments. Ideally, the allocation base correlates service department variable costs directly with units of service department output.

Ambulatory Surgery: Outpatient surgery—a surgical event in which the patient does not stay in the hospital overnight.

Ancillary Charges: Charges for services other than those included in the basic room rate, such as radiology and laboratory tests.

Ancillary Services: Services other than those included in the basic room rate, such as radiology and laboratory tests.

Aspirate: To inhale fluid into the lungs.

Assistant Administrator: A member of the hospital management team that reports to the hospital administrator and often has line responsibility for one or more hospital departments.

Audit Report: An annual report prepared by external certified public accountants on the financial condition of a business institution.

Average Charge per Day: The sum of all hospital charges divided by the number of patient days.

Average Lenght-of-stay: The number of days spent by an average patient in a hospital. The sum of total patient days divided by the total number of admissions.

Beta: The b in the linear regression equation: $Y = a + bX$ or in the multiple regression equation $Y = a + b1X1 + b2X2 + bnXn$. The beta indicates the importance of the effect of the independent variable on the dependent variable.

Billed Charges: The charges a hospital lists for its services and the amount that self-pay patients (e.g. patients without health insurance) pay for hospital goods and services. Insurance companies usually pay a lower amount than billed charges.

Blue Cross: The first prepaid medical care company in the United States.

Break-even: The point at which a business organization neither makes nor loses money.

Business Office Manager: The hospital manager responsible for the creation, management and collection of patient accounts receivable.

Capital Budget: The budget for long-term assets (equipment and facilities).

Capitation Payment: A prospective payment system wherein a hospital or physician receives a fixed monthly payment to provide a specified set of medical services to a person covered for specified healthcare benefits.

Case Management: The process whereby the provision of medical services is managed for maximum positive outcome at the most efficient cost.

Case Mix Adjusted Average Charge: The average charge per patient day divided by the hospital's case mix index.

Case Mix Index: A numerical index developed by HCFA designed to measure the average intensity of care offered by the hospital. A hospital with a case mix index of 1.50, for example, treats patients that require 50 percent more resources in constant dollars on the average than a hospital with a case-mix index of 1.00.

Case Mix: The mix of patient diagnoses treated by a hospital in a calendar year.

Catastrophic Care: An unusually expensive episode of care.

Central Supply: The department that provides medical supplies to hospital departments.

Certificate Of Need: In the 1960s and 1970s some states enacted Certificate of Need Legislation stating that hospitals had to receive a state certificate of approval from a designated central planning organization before acquiring equipment or facilities costing more than $25,000. Those hospitals not receiving certificates of need would not be eligible for cost reimbursement under Medicare.

Charge Master: A list of hospital or physician fees for each service or procedure possible as of a given point in time.

Cholecystectomy: An operation to remove the gall bladder.

Construction Cost Accounting: A branch of cost accounting that accumulates costs by task for construction contractors.

Contingency Pool: A cost center for the accumulation of costs whose probability could not be accurately estimated at the beginning of a construction contract.

Contribution Margin: Revenue minus variable costs.

Controllable Costs: Costs that are easily influenced by a manager—costs a manager can incur, increase, reduce or cancel. Non-controllable costs are those that a manager cannot easily influence.

Controller: The CFO of an organization.

Cost: The cash or cash equivalent value sacrificed for goods and services that are expected to bring a current or future benefit to the organization. Compare with Expense.

Cost Accounting: A branch of accounting concerned with the determination of the cost of services and products manufactured.

Cost Determination: The process of determining the cost of a good or service. The procedure is typically to accumulate product costs including direct labor, direct materials and overhead into a cost pool that is then divided by the number of homogeneous units produced.

Cost Determination Module: In a hospital cost accounting system, the software module that determines product or service costs.

Cost Objective: A function, organizational subdivision, contract or other work unit for which cost data are desired, and for which provision is made to accumulate and measure the costs of contracts, products, etc. Costs are allocated to cost objectives for two reasons: (1) decision making, and (2) control.

Cost Pool: A place where costs are accumulated for a specific objective such as pricing.

Cost Reimbursement: A payment system wherein the hospital receives full costs plus a markup to cover the time value of money and the cost of inflation.

Cost Roll-Up: The accumulation and summation of the costs of primary products to determine the costs of intermediate or final products.

Cost Shifting: The practice of shifting the costs of providing services from one group of patients to another group. Providers of care do this by raising the prices paid by self-pay patients to cover discounts given to insurance companies and shortfalls from Medicare and Medicaid reimbursement. Insurance companies do this by subsidizing the healthcare costs of one block of insured with the premiums of another block.

Cost Variance: The difference between standard and actual costs.

Cost Volume Profit Analysis: An analysis of how total and per-unit product costs change as production volume changes.

Department-Based Cost Accounting: A cost accounting system wherein the smallest cost center is the hospital department. Cost per patient day is usually calculated by summing department costs, then dividing by total patient days. Department-based cost accounting systems do not accumulate and report the costs of individual products and services. Department-based cost accounting systems were the predominant hospital cost accounting system prior to the introduction DRG reimbursement, as more detailed information was not needed under previous payment systems.

Department Head: The manager of a hospital department.

Department Overhead: Indirect costs arising within a hospital department, as contrasted with indirect costs allocated from other hospital departments.

Department Supervisor: The administrative supervisor of a hospital department.

Dependent Variable: In the linear regression equation $Y = a + bX$, Y is the dependent variable, the variable that is influenced by X.

Depreciation: In accounting, an allowance that is established to account for the reduction in the value of property because of wear, deterioration or obsolescence.

Diagnosis Related Group (DRG): A grouping of illnesses, based on diagnosis, procedures performed, age of the patient and discharge status which relate to the same body system and consume about the same amount (cost) of hospital resources. HCFA has established approximately 500 DRGs, each of which has a fixed hospital payment.

Dietary Department: The department responsible for providing patient meals.

Direct Labor: Labor that is easily traceable to a product or service. Compare with Indirect Labor.

Direct Materials: Materials that are easily traceable to a product or service. Compare with Indirect Materials.

Director of Nursing: The supervisor responsible for all nursing departments within the hospital.

Director of Reimbursement: A hospital manager responsible for negotiating contracts with insurance companies, training hospital managers how to make money on those contracts, and managing the contracts.

Disparate Information: Unequal information among the parties to a contract.

Double Apportionment Allocation Method: A method for distributing costs from service departments to revenue-producing departments. The first step is to distribute costs from all service departments to all other service and revenue departments. The second step is the distribution of the resulting department costs using the step-down methodology.

DRG: See *Diagnosis Related Group*.

DRG Cost Accounting System: A hospital cost accounting system with a DRG as the final cost objective.

Economic Order Quantity (EOQ): The optimal quantity of inventory or materials that should be ordered to reduce ordering and inventory costs.

Eighty/Twenty Rule: Eighty percent of a hospital's procedures generate twenty percent of the revenue.

Employee Council: A committee of hospital employees, often elected, whose purpose is to represent the viewpoints and concerns of the employees to management.

Enrollee: One person covered in a health benefit plan.

Epidemiologist: A physician who studies communicable diseases.

Ergonomics: The study of work—more specifically the study of ways the workplace can be improved to minimize employee injury and fatigue.

Expense: An expired cost—a cost that has been recorded on the income statement. Compare with Cost.

Factoring—Accounts Receivable: The sale by a firm of its accounts receivable to an agency at a discount. Because of the cost, firms usually employ factoring with a desperate need for cash.

Fee-for-Service: The traditional process where the insurer or third-party administrator pays one amount for each service, often the full amount billed by the physician or hospital.

Final Cost Objective: A cost objective that has allocated to it both direct and indirect costs. Final cost objectives are used to accumulate the costs of finished products.

Final Product: The final cost objective.

Finance Committee: In a corporation or hospital this is usually a committee of the board. Responsibilities of most finance committees include: (1) reviewing and approving the annual operating and capital budgets, (2) establishing and reviewing relationships with banks, (3) establishing and reviewing financial policies, (4) receiving reports from the internal auditor, and (5) reviewing financial statements.

Financial Accounting: The branch of accounting that is concerned with preparing financial statements for users outside the business (e.g., shareholders, governmental entities, regulators, banks, etc.). Financial accounting is debit-credit oriented, highly structured, rule oriented, and historical. Compare with Management Accounting.

Fixed Labor: Labor that does not change in response to changes in production volume.

Fixed Overhead: Overhead that does not

change in response to changes in production volume.

Fixed-price Contract: A contract whose price has been established in advance of the production of the good or service. The price of a fixed price contract does not change, regardless of the actual cost to the contractor or provider of delivering that good or service.

Fixed-price Reimbursement: A payment system that prospectively determines the price of a good or service prior to the production or delivery of that good or service. Compare with Cost Reimbursement

Flexible Budget. A budget that is responsive to changes in production volume. Flexible budgets usually consist of both fixed and variable costs.

For-Profit Hospital: A hospital that is organized and incorporated to provide a return to shareholders.

Full Cost Accounting: An accounting technique that assigns full costs to products (direct labor, direct materials, variable overhead and fixed overhead). Compare with Variable Cost Accounting.

Functional Cost Center Budgeting: Budgeting by department or function. Compare with Product Line Budgeting.

Gatekeeper Physician: Under an HMO, the physician who must approve all healthcare received by a patient—not just the care provided by the gatekeeper physician herself/herself.

Generic Drugs: A non brand-name drug. These drugs are often manufactured by the same pharmaceutical companies that manufacture the brand name drug, but cost less because (1) research costs have typically been recouped during the patent period, (2) the generic drug is not allocated advertising and marketing costs, and (3) the manufacturer believes it can maximize profits by segmenting the market and selling the same product to different customers at different prices.

Group Model HMO: An HMO in which the physicians are in private group practice and contract to provide physician services to the HMO as a group.

Health Care Financing Administration: The government agency responsible for the administration of the Medicare.

HMO—Group Model: Compare with **HMO—Staff Model.**

HMO—Staff Model: An HMO in which the HMO employs the primary physicians. Payment is often a fixed salary plus a bonus. Compare with HMO—Group Model.

Healthcare Financial Management Association (HFMA): A professional association for accountants and other finance professionals who earn their living in the healthcare industry.

Home Health Care: Services provided by physicians, nurses, physical therapists, certified home healthcare aides, and other professionals in the home (as opposed to an institutional setting). Home healthcare is usually less expensive than institutional care and is receiving increasing attention under prospective payment system payment systems that provide incentives to treat the patient in non-inpatient settings.

Hospital Administrator: The hospital's CEO.

Hospital Overhead: Indirect costs incurred in service departments, and subsequently allocated to revenue departments. In this book we differentiate this from department overhead which, are indirect costs incurred within the specific revenue-producing department.

Inappropriate or Excessive Utilization of Healthcare Services: The demand for or provision of more goods and services (in terms of cost) than necessary to provide the patient with the best possible health outcome.

Incentive Reimbursement: A reimbursement system designed to provide incentives for the healthcare provider (i.e., hospital or physician) to act in the best economic and medical interests of the patient.

Income Multiplier: An economic term used to denote the effect of secondary spending within a community.

Indemnity Insurance Plan: The traditional insurance design that provided few incentives for cost control. Indemnity policies usually (1) have a deductible, (2) pay a percentage of billed charges, (3) have not designated provider network, (4) provide little or no prospective, concurrent, and retrospective review, and (5) pay physicians and hospitals fee-for-service and cost reimbursement.

Independent Variable: In the regression equation $Y = a + bX$, this is the X variable. The Independent Variable influences the behavior of the Y variable (also known as the Dependent Variable).

Indirect Labor: Labor that can't be easily identified with or costed to the product. An example in a manufacturing plant might be the production supervisor. Compare with Direct

Labor.

Indirect Materials: Materials that can't be easily identified with or costed to the product. Compare with Direct Materials.

Industrial Engineer: A person who establishes labor standards for manufacturing production. Industrial engineers often are responsible to find ways to increase efficiency and reduce waste.

Industrial Engineered Standards: See Standard.

Industrial Medicine: A package of services and products provided employers by medical organizations. These services are designed to reduce Workers Compensation costs by (1) decreasing through the use of ergonomics the number of accidents in the work place, (2) reducing employee Workers Compensation fraud, (3) reducing the healthcare costs of legitimate accidents through managed care.

Infections Committee: A hospital committee that monitors in-house infections. The committee is to identify and correct practices causing those infections.

Inpatient Services: Services provided to patients that have been admitted to stay overnight as inpatients to the hospital.

Insurance Premium: A payment made by an employer or enrollee for health insurance.

Intermediary: The middleman between the covered person and the provider. The function of the intermediary is to receive premiums and pay claims to physicians, hospitals and other healthcare providers. In this book, an intermediary may or may not be an insurer. In this book, the term intermediary is used synonymously with the term third-party payer.

Intermediate Product: An intermediate costs objective derived by summing the costs of the primary cost objectives that compose an intermediate cost objective. Intermediate products are not final cost objectives. Intermediate cost objectives are summed to obtain final cost objectives.

Intravenous: Through the vein.

IPA (Independent Practice Association) HMO: A set of independent physicians and other allied health care professionals, whether or not part of a group practice, who have contracted with a third party payer or provider network to provide health care services at other than full cost (charge) basis.

Job Costing: A cost accounting system for unique products (as opposed to process costing for homogeneous products).

Job Evaluation Points: Points used to determine the pay of specific jobs. In theory, these points correlate directly with pay in the marketplace. Job evaluation points are often calculated through regression analysis. In the case study presented, they are the Y in the equation $Y = a + b1X1 + b2X2 + b3X3 + bnXn$.

Joint Conference Committee: A hospital committee composed of members of the medical staff, administration and the governing board. The Joint Conference Committee is coordination between these three bodies.

Labor Cost Variance: The difference between what per unit product labor costs should have been and what they actually were.

Lane: In the compensation study developed in the novel, a salary lane is a grouping of individual jobs, all of which have the same entry point, range, and number of steps.

Lenght-of-stay: The number of consecutive days a patient has stayed overnight in the hospital, counting either the day of admission or the day of discharge but not both.

Life-Flight: An air ambulance service using helicopters and fixed wing aircraft.

Linear Accelerator: Hospital equipment used in the treatment of cancer.

Loan Committee: The bank committee responsible for approving loans to the bank's customers.

Magnetic Resonance Imaging (MRI): A technique used by Radiologists to create an image of internal body structures. MRI images usually provide detail for tissues not well delineated by x-rays.

Managed Care: A philosophy and system of reducing healthcare costs through the management of healthcare by intermediaries or their representatives.

Management Accounting: A division of accounting specializing in the production of information for internal managers (as contrasted with financial accounting that produces information for external users).

Managing Partner: The senior partner in a public accounting firm.

Margin Of Safety: The difference between current sales and break-even sales, assuming current sales exceed break-even sales.

Marginal Costing: A costing system wherein only marginal costs of production comprise product costs. Compare with Variable Cost Accounting and Full Cost Accounting.

Materials Cost Variance: The difference between standard material cost and actual material costs for a unit of product.

Maternity: A catchall term used for the condition of pregnancy and delivery and the associated medical services.

Medicaid: A governmental program funded with state and federal funds to provide healthcare to the indigent.

Medical Director: A physician (often employed by the hospital) who has responsibility for supervising the hospital activities of the medical staff.

Medical Records Department: A department that creates and stores the patient's hospital medical record.

Medicare: A federally funded program to provide healthcare benefits to those sixty-five years of age and older, and certain under-age-65 disabled individuals.

Milestone—Construction Accounting: A signal indicating that a predefined task or series of tasks have been finished. Unlike tasks, milestones do not consume resources. They are, in a sense, "road markers" that indicate project progress.

Mixed Costs: Costs that have fixed and variable components.

Net Present Value: The difference between the present value of the cash outflows and case inflows of a project for a given period.

Nonprofit Organization: An organization formed to provide services that are often not available through the private sector. Surpluses of nonprofit organizations cannot inure to the benefit of specific persons.

Normal Cost Accounting: A cost accounting systems that defines product cost as the sum of direct labor, direct material and overhead applied. Compare with Standard Cost Accounting and Actual Cost Accounting.

Normal Delivery: A noncomplicated vaginal or c-section delivery of a baby.

Not-for-Profit Organization: In this book this term is used synonymously with the term non-profit organization, although under the tax code there are certain technical differences.

Nurse Practitioner: A registered nurse who has received additional training and is licensed to perform predefined diagnostic and treatment services previously reserved for physicians.

Occupancy Rate: The percent of hospitals beds occupied.

Occupational Medicine: See Industrial Medicine.

Oncology: The study of tumors.

Opportunity Cost: The sacrificed benefit when choosing one alternative versus another alternative.

Outpatient Services: Services provided by hospital departments to patients not admitted to the hospital for an overnight stay.

Outpatient Surgery: Surgery performed on patients who have not been admitted to the hospital for an overnight stay. Synonymous with ambulatory surgery.

Over-Capacity: In terms of facilities or equipment, more capacity than needed to meet current or near-term demand.

Overhead: Indirect product costs.

Overhead Allocation: The process of allocating service department indirect costs to revenue departments, or service and department indirect costs to cost objectives.

Overhead Cost Variance: The difference between the standard overhead costs of a product and actual overhead costs.

Patient Day: One day spent by an inpatient in the hospital.

Per-Admission Payment: A prospective payment system wherein the hospital is paid a fixed price for a hospital admission, regardless of the actual cost of the goods and services rendered to the patient.

Per-Diem Payment: A prospective payment system wherein the hospital is paid a fixed price per patient day, regardless of the actual cost of goods and services rendered to the patient each day.

Performance Reporting—Functional Level: Performance reporting on hospital departments.

Performance Reporting—Product Level: Performance reporting by product.

Physical Therapy: The treatment of musculoskeletal disease, injury, etc., by physical means. Physical therapy can include massage, infrared or ultraviolet light, electrotherapy, hydrotherapy, heat or exercise.

Physician Hospital Organization: An organization of physicians and one or more hospitals that contracts with insurance companies or employers to provide medical care, often with acceptance of risk.

Practice Protocols: Written procedures for

handling specific medical conditions or performing medical services.

Precertification: A process wherein a patient or provider receives permission from the insurer or managed care entity for a medical service in advance of the provision of that service. Services not precertified where precertification is required may not be reimbursed in full, or at all, by insurance companies.

Preferred Provider Organization (PPO): A group of physicians who contracts with an intermediary to provide medical services using a billing mechanism other than billed charges. Preferred Provider Organizations are designed to manage care without capitation payment or the employment of physicians by HMOs. The term PPO is also sometimes used to refer to the insurance product provided by the Preferred Provider Organization.

Premium: See Insurance Premium.

Prenatal Care: Care received by the mother and child, prior to the birth of the child.

President of Medical Staff: An elected officer of the medical staff who represents the medical staff to administration and the governing board.

Preventive Medicine: Medical goods and services designed to prevent or diagnose (as opposed to treat) illnesses.

Price Elasticity: An economic term referring to a condition in which the demand for a product is directly influenced by price.

Primary Care Hospital: A hospital that provides the broad spectrum of primary inpatient goods and services for patients who do not need highly specialized healthcare services. Other classifications include Secondary Care Hospitals and Tertiary Care Hospitals.

Primary Product: A primary cost objective.

Procedure: A medical test, service or surgery provided by a healthcare provider. In this novel, procedures are a primary cost objective in the cost accounting system designed for the Peter Brannan Community Hospital.

Process Costing: A costing system used to cost homogeneous products (as opposed to job costing, which is used to cost unique one of a kind products).

Product Based Cost Accounting: A cost accounting system whose cost objective is the product (as opposed to the hospital department).

Prospective payment system: A payment system wherein prices are set prior to the provision of medical goods and services.

Radiology: A branch of science dealing with the use of radiant sources energy (especially x-rays) and its uses as in the diagnosis and treatment of disease by x-rays.

Rate Review: In this novel this refers to a process mandated by law wherein hospitals must receive approval in advance for changes in hospital rates.

Ratio of costs to charges (RCC): A methodology traditionally used by hospitals to determine procedure costs.

Reagent: A substance used in the laboratory to detect or measure another substance.

Regression Analysis: A statistical tool that establishes the relationship between a dependent variable and one or more independent variables.

Reimbursement: A methodology whereby a provider is paid for services, supplies or accommodations provided.

Relative Value Unit (RVU): A measure of resource consumption

Relevant Costs: Costs that are useful for the **cost decision at hand.**

Residency: The segment of the physician's training that traditionally takes place after medical school, and after the internship. Residencies prepare physicians for specialties.

Resource Based Relative Value System (RBRVS): The payment system used by Medicare for outpatient physician reimbursement. The system is basically a relative value unit (RVU) scale. Resource inputs include: (1) total work input performed by the physician for each service, (2) practice costs including overhead and insurance premiums, and (3) the cost of specialty training. One criticism of the system is that it does not include a measurement factor for the improvement in the health of the patient.

Retrospective Reimbursement: A payment system wherein the payment is determined after the provision of medical goods and services.

Return on Investment (ROI): A measurement used to determine the financial attractiveness of an **investment opportunity.**

Revenue Department: A hospital department that earns revenue. Revenue departments include nursing, radiology, laboratory, physical therapy, respiratory therapy, emergency center, cafeteria, etc.

Richness Index: A measurement system used to compare the benefit values of different health employee benefit plan designs.

Room Rate: A daily charge by the hospital designed to cover basic nursing and bed and board services. Total charges comprise room rate and ancillary service charges.

Salary Lane: See Lane.

Salary Step: A fixed percentage increment in a salary lane designed to pay the employee for productivity gained through experience.

Secondary Care Hospital: A hospital that provides more specialized care than a primary care hospital, but less specialized care than a tertiary care hospital.

Self-Pay Patients: Patients who are responsible for their own healthcare bill (i.e., patients who do not have health insurance).

Service Department: Hospital departments that provide services to revenue producing departments and do not generate revenue themselves. Service departments in a hospital include administration, housekeeping, laundry, business office, grounds, maintenance, etc.

Staff Model HMO: An HMO that employs its medical staff.

Stakeholder: An person who has a financial or other interest in an organization, project or concept.

Standard Cost: What a product should cost (versus what it actually costs). In cost accounting standards are commonly established for product direct labor, direct materials, and fixed and variable overhead.

Standard Cost Accounting System: A costing system that assigns standard versus actual direct labor, materials and overhead to products. Compare with Actual Cost Accounting System and Normal Cost Accounting System.

Step-Down Methodology Of Cost Allocation: A method of allocating service department costs to revenue departments.

Sunk Cost: A cost incurred that cannot be changed or recovered.

Task, Construction Accounting: An undertaking involving work or difficulty. Tasks consume labor, materials and overhead.

Tertiary Care Hospital: A hospital that provides a high degree of specialized care. See Primary Care Hospital and Secondary Care Hospital

Third Party Administrator: See Intermediary

Third Party Payer: See Intermediary

Traditional Insurance Program: See Indemnity Insurance Plan

Treatment Protocols: Written procedures for handling specific medical conditions or performing medical services.

Underwrite: In insurance, to assume liability for a specified sum in the event of a named loss or damage, or in healthcare, the incurral of a healthcare cost.

Utilization Review: Retrospective review for medical appropriateness of medical services received by a patient.

Variable Cost Accounting (Variable Costing): A cost accounting methodology that assigns only variable costs to products. Compare with Full Cost Accounting.

Variable Labor: Labor that increases in volume as production volume increases.

Variance: In cost accounting, the difference between what a product should cost and what it actually cost.

Working Capital: In accounting, the excess of readily convertible assets over current liabilities.

Y-Intercept: On an X/Y graph the point where the regression line intercepts the Y-axis. When the regression equation $Y = a + bX$ is used as a cost function, the Y intercept represents fixed costs, and is the point (0,a).

Appendix Three

Abbreviations

AHA   American Healthcare Association

AHS   American Hospital Supply

CAS   Cost accounting system

APGS   Medicare's ambulatory classification or grouping system

CCU   Coronary care unit

CEO   Chief executive officer

CFO   Chief financial officer

CNO   Chief nursing officer

CVP   Cost-volume-profit

DME   Durable medical equipment

DRG   Diagnosis related group

E&Y   Ernst & Young, LLP

EC   Emergency Center

EOQ   Economic order quantity

FTE   Full time equivalent

GIGO   Garbage-in-garbage-out

HCFA   Health Care Financing Administration

HFMA   Healthcare Financial Management Association

HMO   Health maintenance organization

ICDA-8   International Classification of Diseases Amended Version Eight

ICDA-9   International Classification of Diseases Amended Version Nine

ICU   Intensive care unit

IRR   Internal rate of return

IV   Intravenous

JCAHO   Joint Commission on Accreditation of Healthcare Organizations

JIT   Just-in-time

MRI   Magnetic resonance imaging

O.B.	Obstetrics
O.R.	Operating room
PHO	Physician Hospital Organization
PPO	Preferred Provider Organization
PT	Physical Therapy
RBC	Red blood count
RBRVS	Resource based relative value system.
RCC	Ratio of costs to charges
ROI	Return on investment
RVU	Relative value unit
TPA	Third-party administrator
TQM	Total quality management
WBC	White blood count

Order Information

Additional copies can be ordered through Traemus Books.

January 1, 2003 Retail: $24.95 plus shipping. Bookstores, 25% discount off of retail price (bookstore price $18.71)

For additional information or to order by phone call: 1-801-525-9643

To order through the Internet visit: http:// www.traemus-books.com

We accept Visa

To order with a purchase order, mail your purchase order to:

Traemus Books

2481 West 1425 South

Syracuse, UT 84075

Or

Fax your purchase order to 801-773-7669

Email authors at kevin_stocks@byu.edu

Volume discounts are available.